INTERSCIENCE MONOGRAPHS
ON CHEMISTRY

Interscience Monographs on Chemistry

INORGANIC CHEMISTRY SECTION

Edited by F. Albert Cotton and G. Wilkinson

Other Volumes to follow

ISOCYANIDE COMPLEXES OF METALS

L. MALATESTA

Professor of Chemistry,
University of Milan, Italy
S.c. Accademia Naz. dei Lincei

F. BONATI

Associate Professor,
University of Milan, Italy

1969
A WILEY–INTERSCIENCE PUBLICATION

John Wiley & Sons Ltd.
London   New York   Sydney   Toronto

547.05
m 29 i
71310
Sept., 1970

Made and printed in Great Britain by
William Clowes and Sons, Limited, London and Beccles

PREFACE

The present book has its origin in the review which appeared under the same title in the first volume of the well known *Progress in Inorganic Chemistry*, published by John Wiley. During the time that has elapsed since 1958, when the review was written, much more material has accumulated. In particular, structural and some other physical data have been collected, and a few problems solved, while other questions (*e.g.* the reactivity of oxygen and other small molecules with zerovalent isocyanide metal complexes) are only in the initial phase of study.

We believe that interest in this field will go on growing steadily, for the isocyanide complexes of metals are suitable material for new preparative work, using the now very rich arsenal of modern physicochemical methods in theoretical speculations, and, last but not least, in problems of catalysis.

We wish to express our warmest thanks to Professor F. A. Cotton, who carefully read nearly all of our typescript.

L. MALATESTA
F. BONATI

v

CONTENTS

1 SURVEY OF THE PROPERTIES OF ISOCYANIDES

STRUCTURE OF ISOCYANIDES

No x-ray structure of a free isocyanide is known. A few x-ray structures of complexes with isocyanides as ligands are known, but these data cannot be applied to the free ligand since complex formation must surely alter the structure of the ligand, at least in principle.

Two structures were proposed in the old literature, one by Nef[1,2] (1) and the other by Langmuir[3] (2):

$$N\!\!=\!\!C: \qquad R\!\!-\!\!\overset{\oplus}{N}\!\!\equiv\!\!\overset{\ominus}{C}:$$
$$R\diagup$$

$$(1) \qquad\qquad (2)$$

The prevalence of the canonical structure (2) was ascertained rather early, owing to the parachor value of isocyanide (66 units)[4,5].

The absence of a measurable electric dipole moment in 1,4-diisocyanobenzene[6] suggested that the isocyano groups form an angle of 180° with the axis of the benzene ring passing through the 1 and 4 positions.

Electron diffraction data on methyl isocyanide at first suggested that the R—N—C angle might be anything between 160 and 180°[7]. This value and the accompanying NC distance (1·18 Å), intermediate between the value required by a simple double bond (1·262 Å) and that required by a triple bond (1·150 Å), led Pauling[8] to suggest that the contribution of structure 1 might be anything up to 26%. More recent results by microwave spectroscopy, reported in Table 2.2 with other data, have shown that, by symmetry, the R—N—C angle in CH_3NC must be 180°[9]. This result suggests that here, as in the complexed isocyanide molecules, the simple valence-bond theory should be superseded by the molecular-orbital theory. According to the latter, the R—N—C angle must be 180°; what is generally described in valence-bond terminology as 'a higher contribution of form 2 over form 1,' to explain, for example, the spectroscopic properties of hydrogen-bonded isocyanide, can be viewed as a different distribution of electronic density in the two π and one σ orbitals between carbon and nitrogen.

PREPARATION OF ISOCYANIDES

Isocyanides, also often called alkyl or aryl isonitriles and carbylamines, can be considered to be derived from the tautomeric form of hydrogen cyanide. The hypothetical hydrogen isocyanide has never been isolated as such, although its infrared spectrum in an argon matrix has been recorded (Table 1.1). Recently it was found possible to isolate complexes, such as $HNCM(CO)_5$ (M = Cr, Mo, W), where hydrogen isocyanide is stabilized through coordination to a metal[10].

The preparation of isocyanides was not very satisfactory up to recent times but now, in addition to the classical methods of

Gautier[11,12] and Hofmann[13,14], other synthetic procedures are available. Moreover, because of industrial interest in isonitriles, a great many bi- or polyfunctional isocyanides are known, including synthetic xanthocilline, a naturally occurring antibiotic. (A list of isocyanides is given in Tables 1.2, 1.3 and 1.4). The principal synthetic routes will now be described.

Dehydration of *N*-monosubstituted formamides, RNHCHO

This method of preparation is rather general and has been used for preparing a great many isocyanides, both aliphatic and aromatic, with or without additional functional groups. The formation of a trace of isocyanide by pyrolysis of *N*-substituted formamide had been observed by Nef in 1892[1,2], but the potentialities of the reaction were exploited only in the late fifties by Ugi[15,16], who found the conditions required for obtaining good yields and a wide number of compounds. A typical Ugi reaction[17], e.g.

$$RNH(CHO) + COCl_2 + 2 R_3'N \rightarrow RNC + CO_2 + 2 R_3'N.HCl$$

is generally carried out in a polar solvent, such as a chlorinated hydrocarbon. As dehydrating agents, a large number of compounds were successfully used; they include phosgene[17,18,19,20], cyanuric chloride[21], phosphorous (III) halide, phosphorous oxyhalides[16,20,22], thionyl chloride and *p*-toluenesulphonyl chloride[15]. In all cases the presence of a base is required: tertiary amines (triethylamine, pyridine, quinoline), alkaline carbonates, potassium *t*-butoxide and even liquid ammonia[23] have been used. The related *N*-monosubstituted thioformamides give the same reaction[24].

As examples to illustrate this method and some of its modifications the preparations of some isocyanides are reported in the Appendix.

Reaction of an organic compound with a cyanide

This method was used by Gautier in 1869[11,12]. Until recently it was the preferred method for preparing aliphatic isonitriles. The general reaction is:

$$R—X + AgCN \rightarrow R—NC.AgX \xrightarrow{KCN} R—NC + KAg(CN)_2 + KX$$

Only traces of isonitrile are obtained with alkaline cyanides, while transition-metal cyanides afford a variable mixture of the two isomers. The best conditions for the production of alkyl isonitriles require the use of silver cyanide: the preparation of ethyl isonitrile by this method is described in *Organic Syntheses*[25]. Nevertheless, the reaction of silver cyanide with a reactive halide does not necessarily afford an isocyanide, rather than a nitrile. Indeed, treatment of trimethylsilyl chloride with silver cyanide gave trimethylsilyl cyanide[26].

Quite recently a novel way of preparing aliphatic isocyanides was discovered. By reaction of an olefin, hydrogen cyanide and cuprous bromide, isonitrile copper (I) complexes were produced, e.g. $(Me_3CNC)_3CuBr$ or $(Me_3CNC)CuCN$; decomposition of the complexes with aqueous KCN afforded the isonitrile. It was realized that the olefins must have a disubstituted olefinic carbon (RR′C:) for the *N*-alkylation reaction; probably the driving force of this unusual reaction is the formation of the copper complex (see p. 40).

Carbylamine reaction

$$R—NH_2 + CHCl_3 + 3 KOH \rightarrow R—NC + 3 KCl + 3 H_2O$$

Aromatic isocyanides were often prepared by this method, in its original version due to Hofmann[13,14] or in a subsequent improvement[27]. The method can also be used for aliphatic isonitriles, except for the lowest members: but no advantage on the other methods is gained. Bifunctional isocyanides can be prepared, such as β-dialkylaminoethyl isonitrile[28] or *p*-isocyanobenzoic acid[29]. Generally, the yields are not very high: around 20% with alcoholic potassium hydroxide and around 45% with solid potassium hydroxide. Higher yields were reported in the literature, but they are probably due to the presence of unreacted amine in the distillate[17,30]. However, the presence of a trace of unreacted aniline in phenyl isonitrile was shown to be effective in preventing a quick polymerization to blue indigo-dianil[31]. Removal of contaminant amine by a zinc salt was described by Sacco[32].

Other modifications of the reaction involve the thermal decomposition of sodium trichloroacetate in the presence of aryl amines: a dark tar (and sometimes only tar) is always present owing to the need for elevated temperatures[33]. A way of overcoming this disadvantage in the preparation of aromatic isonitriles has recently been reported[34]. To a toluene–hexane solution of an aromatic primary amine (0·2 mole) and sodium *tert*-butoxide (0·6 mole), chloroform was added drop by drop at 0–5°. After 5 hours' standing the mixture was fractionated to afford the isonitrile. Phenyl, *o*- and *p*-tolyl, *o*- and *p*-chloro-phenylisocyanide were prepared in 71–98% yields.

A Russian paper[35] gives details on the preparation of butyl isocyanide in moderate yields from butylamine, carbon tetrachloride and sodium.

Isocyanides by reduction

It is possible to obtain moderate yields of phenyl or *p*-chlorophenyl isonitrile by treatment of $ArN:CCl_2$ with triphenyl- or tributyl-phosphine, neat or in petroleum ether[36]. Deoxygenation of isocyan-ates or desulphurization of isothiocyanates has also been reported, employing tertiary phosphites[37] or 2-phenyl-3-methyl-1,3,2-oxaza-phospholidine[38]. The loss of oxygen or of sulphur can also take place during the reaction of isocyanate or isothiocyanate with metal carbonyls to give the isonitrile complexes[39].

Other reducing agents which have been employed for this purpose include Et_3P[40], copper[41], triphenyltin hydride[42] and methyl lithium[43]. Photolytic reduction is also possible[44].

Miscellaneous preparations

Dehydration of aldoximes[45,46] with methyl ketene acetals or with *p*-toluenesulphonyl chloride[47], opening of the ring of certain heterocycles and other reactions give rise to some isocyanide, often with substantial quantities of nitrile, so that these methods do not have general validity. A review of these and other methods for the formation of isonitriles, as well as of reaction mechanisms, is available[17].

Another synthetic approach leading directly to isocyanide com-plexes, which are in turn sources of isocyanides, is the alkylation of cyano-complexes, and this has been used repeatedly; the most recent work on the subject is due to Heldt[48].

CHEMICAL PROPERTIES

Alkyl isocyanides are colourless liquids, somewhat more volatile than the corresponding nitriles; the difference in the boiling points of the lowest members of the series is about 20°c. They have penetrating and disgusting odours, which are very useful for detecting even traces of compound; they were assumed to be extremely toxic, because of their ability to combine with haemoglobin[49,50,51]. Recent evidence showed, however, that they are not especially toxic to warm-blooded animals. Doses of 500–5000 mg/Kg were tolerated by mice, either orally or subcutaneously[52].

Isocyanides are highly reactive. They polymerize easily and above 200–250° they rearrange to cyanides, the rearrangement being accompanied by some polymerization. The isocyanide to cyanide thermal isomerization was studied recently[53]. A series of aryl and alkyl isocyanides was investigated at a reaction temperature of 200°c. The unimolecular, first-order thermal isomerization goes through essentially synchronous bond-breaking and bond-making, and little charge separation develops in the transition state. Indeed, the stereochemical configuration at the migrating carbon atom is retained, the carbon skeleton does not rearrange in the isomerization of cyclobutyl isocyanide and the reaction rate is not much affected by variations of the *para* substituents in aryl isocyanides.

The thermal isomerization of other isocyanides was also studied. Recent data are available for methyl isocyanide and deuterated methyl isocyanide[54,55,57], phenyl isocyanide[58], *p*-tolyl isocyanide[59] and even some isocyanide derivatives of 5-α-cholestane[60], with retention of configuration.

Thermal isomerization has also been effected by irradiating methyl isocyanide with radiation having $\lambda = 2537$ Å[61].

Isocyanides are attacked by aqueous acid, according to the following equation[12]:

$$R—NC + HCl + H_2O \rightarrow R—NH_2 . HCl + HCOOH$$

The rate of hydration of *t*-butyl isocyanide has been followed kinetically. The reaction, which is subject to general acid catalysis, involves a rate-determining proton-transfer step[62].

Isocyanides are polymerized rather easily by anhydrous acid or by some transition-metal salts, e.g. nickel (II), cobalt (II) and palladium (II)[63,64]. A small quantity of aniline or hydrazine generally inhibits polymerization of isocyanides. This was evident in the case of phenyl isocyanide, which gives brown tars and blue indigodianil on short standing, even at 20°c, in the absence of these inhibiting compounds. Isolation of a dimer of phenyl isocyanide had been claimed, but the compound was found to be N,N'-diphenylformamidine, formed owing to the presence of aniline in the isocyanide[31].

Isocyanides are stable to alkalies under mild conditions except the first member which undergoes a slow hydrolysis. The rather sensitive vinyl isocyanide, for example, was obtained by action of 10% ethanolic potassium hydroxide on 2-isocyanoethylbenzen-sulphonate[65].

Isocyanides are strong reducing agents. However, they can act as oxidants toward such compounds as Li_2Bipy, or $Li[V(Bipy)_3]$ (Bipy = 2,2'-dipyridyl)[56]. The behaviour of isocyanides at the dropping mercury electrode has been reported, but no conclusions were reached[95]. A review on the organic reactions of isocyanides is available[66].

INFRARED SPECTRA

The infrared and Raman spectra of isocyanides are characterized by a strong CN stretching absorption in the 2100–2200 cm^{-1} region, as required by a bond with high bond order. The actual values of the CN stretching frequency are not greatly sensitive to the solvent (see Table 1.5)[67,68,69].

The value of the CN absorption band of isocyanide is approximately 100 cm^{-1} lower than the corresponding value for a nitrile. A similar difference of approximately 20 cm^{-1} can be found between aliphatic and aromatic isocyanides, as well as nitriles.

The lower value of $\nu(CN)$ for aromatic isocyanides reflects the known ability of the benzene ring to stabilize structures as

There is also a remarkable difference between the intensity of the $\nu(CN)$ band of isocyanides and nitriles[68]. The measured intensity in CCl_4 is 1.46×10^4 mol^{-1} l cm^{-2} for phenyl isocyanide, 0.97×10^4 for n-propyl isocyanide, but 2.1×10^3 and 6×10^2 for benzonitrile and n-propionitrile respectively; parallel values were measured in chloroform and in pentachloro-ethane.

The greater intensity of the isocyanide band compared to that of the nitrile bond is due to the greater charge separation ($-\overset{\oplus}{N}\equiv\overset{\ominus}{C}$) in the former than in the latter compounds. Similarly, electron-attracting substituents in aromatic isocyanides lower $\nu(CN)$ and increase the intensity of the band, while the opposite is true with nitriles[70,71].

The effect on the infrared spectrum of solvents capable of giving hydrogen bonding has been studied. The results of Gillis and Occolowitz[68] showed that the intensity of $\nu(CN)$ in $CHCl_3$ and C_2HCl_5

decreased slightly and the frequency increased (< 10 cm^{-1}) compared with the values recorded for a solution in carbon tetrachloride. The changes were in the opposite direction to those recorded for hydrogen bonds in carbonyl groups[72]. The difference is due to the fact that hydrogen bonding to the carbonyl group increases the single-bond character and the charge separation:

$$\diagdown_{\diagup} C{=}O\cdots H{-}X \leftrightarrow \diagdown_{\diagup} \overset{\delta+}{C}{-}\overset{\centerdot}{O}{-}H\cdots\overset{\delta-}{X}$$

while for the isocyanide group, hydrogen bonding increases the triple bond character and decreases the charge separation:

$$R{-}\overset{\oplus}{N}{\equiv}\overset{\ominus}{C}\cdots HX \leftrightarrow R{-}\overset{\delta+}{N}{\equiv}\overset{\centerdot}{C}{-}H\cdots\overset{\delta-}{X}$$

These results are in agreement with those of Horrocks[67]. The possibility that hydrogen bonding with isocyanide might involve the nitrogen instead of the carbon atom was ruled out by Ferstandig[73,74] and Allerhand[75,76], using alcohols, phenols and phenylacetylene, by i.r. and n.m.r. techniques. All this evidence shows that isocyanides are hydrogen-bonding bases.

NUCLEAR MAGNETIC RESONANCE SPECTRA

The proton n.m.r. spectra of isocyanides show a remarkable characteristic, namely, long range ^{14}N–^{1}H coupling. This has been observed on aliphatic isocyanides[77] and benzyl isocyanide[78]; the numerical value is a few cycles. This coupling, absent in the related nitriles, indicates that the electric-field gradient is unusually small and that the spin–lattice relaxation time of ^{14}N must be comparable to the times associated with the coupling constants. The only other organic nitrogen compounds where similar spin–spin splitting can be observed are some highly symmetrical tetramethylammonium halides.

The absence of ^{14}N–^{1}H spin coupling in the various methylcyanosilanes was taken as evidence against their formulation as methyl-(isocyano)silanes[26].

An ^{1}H–^{1}H decoupling experiment demonstrated that the signs of the spin coupling $J(^{14}$N–^{1}H$_{CH_2})$ and $J(^{14}$N–^{1}H$_{CH_3})$ in ethyl isocyanide are opposite[79].

Formation of a complex generally introduces an electric-field gradient about the ^{14}N nucleus. Consequently the spin–spin splitting is generally absent, with the exception of $(CH_3)_3B.CNCH_3$, for which a highly symmetrical structure was therefore assumed[80].

N.m.r. spectra for ^{14}N are also available[81]. The chemical shift found is quite different from that of nitriles (Table 1.7).

OTHER DATA

Ultraviolet spectra for various isocyanides were reported mainly by Ugi[20]. The isolated isocyano group is not a chromophore; therefore only weak absorption could be found in aliphatic and cyclohexyl isocyanides. However, the CN— group interacts strongly with groups capable of resonance. When it is near to an aromatic group there is a strong increase in the benzenoid absorption band and a red shift if an electron-attracting or releasing substituent is present on the ring.

Mass spectra were recorded for some aliphatic isocyanides together with those of the corresponding nitriles[82]. It was found that β-bond cleavage is the principal mode of fragmentation in the isocyanides. In addition, α-bond cleavage is very noticeable here, while it is of minor importance with cyanides. The appearance potentials of the molecular ions were also determined for both isomers. In the methyl and ethyl pairs the ionization potential of the isocyanide is smaller.

While removal of one electron requires 0·6 eV less in isocyanide than in nitrile, it is not possible to state whether it comes from the bonding electrons or from the lone pair.

Details on the gas-chromatographic detection of isocyanides can be found in several places[53,83], including a paper with the stress on the column material[84].

Isocyanide bond refraction, not previously available, was published by Gillis[85]. The bond-refraction coefficients, 28·55 for isocyanides and 29·91 for nitriles, are significantly different.

A new value of dipole moment for the isocyano group bonded to an aromatic carbon was determined recently as 3·44 Debye, against 3·92 for the nitrile group[86]. The value is in fair agreement with the values reported by Sutton for ethyl isocyanide[6] (3·47 D) and phenyl isocyanide (3·49 D).

Some structural data are available, e.g. for CH_3NC, and are given in Table 2.2.

APPENDIX

Preparation of some isocyanides

Methyl isocyanide[83]

N-methylformamide (0·25 mole) was added dropwise in a 10-minute period to a stirred solution of p-tosyl chloride (0·38 mole) and quinoline (1·00 mole) at 75°/60 mm.

Methyl isocyanide distilled rapidly and was collected in a receiver cooled by liquid nitrogen. The purity of the compound (0·13 mole) was found to be 99% according to gas chromatography (propylene glycol-firebrick; 2 m.; 75°; retention volume, 55 ml of helium).

Similar procedures were employed to prepare ∼ 98% pure ethyl, sec-butyl and cyclobutyl isocyanide, all with good yields[83]. For all these the difference between the boiling point of the isocyanide and that of the solvent, isoquinoline, was large enough to allow both a clean separation and the escape of the isocyanide before secondary reactions set in. The reaction can be carried out in a standard vacuum line apparatus.

tert-Butyl isocyanide[17]

Phosgene (caution!) (10·1 mole) is delivered into a stirred solution of N-tert-butyl formamide (10·0 mole) and tributylamine (5·4 l) in 1,3,5-trichlorobenzene (2·5 l) at 10–20°c. After introduction of ammonia (50 g) the reaction product was distilled on a bath at 80–85° and under a pressure of 120–150 Torr and then fractionated. Yield: 648 g or 78%.

Large scale modifications of the above procedure are given[17] together with the detailed preparations of an additional fourteen isonitriles.

Cyclohexyl isocyanide[17]

Phosgene (caution!) is bubbled at a rate of 0·3–0·4 Kg/hour through a solution of N-cyclohexyl formamide (10·0 mole) and triethylamine (3·2 l) in dichloromethane (4·5 l). The rate of bubbling should be such that the solution is kept boiling under reflux. When the boiling stops (after approximately 1·04 Kg of phosgene) the mixture is cooled to 20°c. Then ammonia (400 g) is delivered into the reaction mixture for 1–2 hours. After filtration and concentration to small volume, the residue is distilled. Yield: 955 g or 88%. A modification of this preparation is available in *Organic Synthesis*[19].

Phenyl, benzyl, *o*- and *p*-tolyl isocyanides

The required formylamine (0·200 mole) is dissolved in triethyl-amine (65 ml) and methylene chloride (200 ml). Phosgene (caution!) (0·200 mole) is bubbled into the stirred and ice-cooled mixture. A saturated aqueous solution of sodium carbonate is then added (50 ml) and the organic phase dried over powdered KOH. The compound is isolated by fractional distillation. Yields: 76, 82, 54 and 72% respectively.

An alternative preparation is available for these aromatic isocyan-ides[20]. Potassium *tert*-butoxide (from 0·3 g potassium and 140 ml absolute butanol) is treated with finely powdered formylamine (0·10 mole). To the solution phosphorous oxychloride (0·066 mole) is added dropwise for 5 minutes, while stirring and cooling with ice. Stirring is continued while the mixture is heated for 5 minutes at 40–50°c. Solid carbon dioxide is added (10 g) and everything is poured into a mixture of ice and water (750 ml). The oily isocyanide is extracted with petroleum ether and the extract is combined with those of the aqueous phase (100–150 ml in all). After washing with water and drying over sodium sulphate, the product is fractionated.

According to this alternative procedure, good yields of benzyl, phenyl, *o*- and *p*-tolyl, *p*-methoxyphenyl, *p*-diethylaminophenyl, 2,6-dimethylphenyl, 6-chloro-2-methylphenyl, 2,4,6-trimethylphenyl and 2-naphthyl isocyanides were obtained[20].

Table 1.1   Infrared absorption and force constants of isohydrocyanic and hydrocyanic acid

			$f(HC)$	$f(CN)$	f^1	d	Note	Ref.
HNC	2032	535	3583	7·01	16·45	0·06	0·11	Argon matrix	88
DNC	1940	413	2733	—	—	—	—	Argon matrix	88, 90
HCN	2097	712	3311	5·82	18·02	0·00	0·20	Gaseous state	89, 91

Table 1.2   Aliphatic isocyanides

Compound	B.p.	ν(CN)	Note	Ref.
CH_3—NC	25–30/150 (m.p. − 45°)	2170 (gas) 2157·5 (cetane)	IR spectrum and thermodynamic properties[92]; force constants[93]; Org. Synth.[112]	17, 53 83, 94
C_2H_5—NC	32–35/120 80–82	2148 (cetane) 2151 (gas)	Org. Synth.[25]	17, 53, 83 38, 94
CH_2=CH—NC	45–47	2130	ν (C≡C) : 1613	65
n-C_3H_7—NC	99·5/760	—	—	Beilstein
i-C_3H_7—NC	87–88/730	2140	—	20, 53, 83
n-C_4H_9—NC	40–42/11 116–117/730	2127 (gas)	—	17, 20
i-C_4H_9—NC	—	2125 (gas)	—	83
s-C_4H_9—NC	110–111	2125 (CCl_4)	—	53
t-C_4H_9—NC	92–93/750 60–63/314 37–39/6	2143 (C_6H_{12}) 2127 (CCl_4)	Cf. Table 1.5	17, 53, 94 96, 97

Table 1.2 (*continued*)

Compound	B.p.	ν(CN)	Note	Ref.
n-C_6H_{13}	168–169	—	—	30
n-C_8H_{17}	89–91/12	—	—	30
cyclobutyl isocyanide	—	2137 (gas)	—	83
cyclohexyl isocyanide	62–67/13	2138	U.v. spectrum[20]; *Org. Synth.*[18]	17, 18
1-cyclohexenyl isocyanide	56–59/12	—	—	17, 98
	m.p. 36–38			
$(C_2H_5)_2N(CH_2)_3NC$	40–42/0·04	—	—	17, 28
	105–107/45	—	—	
$(C_2H_5)_2N(CH_2)_2NC$	94–95/45	2100	—	28
$(C_2H_5)_2N-NC$	39/16	—	easily decomposed	99
$(C_2H_5O)_2P(O)OCH_2CH_2NC$	70–71/0·03	—	—	100
$EtOOCCH_2NC$	30–40/15	—	—	97

Table 1.3   Aromatic isocyanides

Compound	M.p.	B.p.	ν(CN)	Note[a]	Ref.
phenyl isocyanide	—	76–78/27, 50–51/11	2117, 2127 (cetane), 2132·5 (CHCl$_3$)	U.v. spectrum	17, 38
o-tolyl isocyanide	—	36–38/0·6, 62–64/11	2122	U.v. spectrum	19, 20, 101
p-tolyl isocyanide	19–20	70–72/8	2125	Influence of the solvent on ν(CN) see Table 1.5; Org. Synth.[19]	33, 102
p-cyanotolyl isocyanide	130 (dec.)	—	2120 (C$_6$H$_{12}$)	U.v. spectrum	17, 67
o-chlorophenyl isocyanide	26–28	58–59/1	2116	U.v. spectrum	20
p-chlorophenyl isocyanide	72–73	61–64/1	2116	U.v. spectrum	20
m-nitrophenyl isocyanide	97–99	—	2120	U.v. spectrum	20
p-nitrophenyl isocyanide	119–120	—	2116	U.v. spectrum	17, 20
o-methoxyphenyl isocyanide	—	65/12	—	—	22
p-methoxyphenyl isocyanide	61–62, 28–29	76–77/1	2125	U.v. spectrum	22, 103
p-hydroxyphenyl isocyanide	87–88	—	—	—	47
p-carboxyphenyl isocyanide	300	—	2130	Cream coloured	29

Table 1.3 (*continued*)

Compound	M.p.	B.p.	ν(CN)	Note[a]	Ref.
p-dimethylaminophenyl isocyanide	53–54	95–98/0.05	2124	U.v. spectrum	20
mesityl isocyanide	42–43	69–71/1	2109	U.v. spectrum	20
2,4,6-trichlorophenyl isocyanide	134–136	—	—	—	104
pentamethylphenyl isocyanide	127–128	—	—	—	17
pentachlorophenyl isocyanide	188–191	—	—	—	17
α-naphthyl isocyanide	—	90–95/0.05	—	—	17
β-naphthyl isocyanide	59–60	100–102/1	2122	U.v. spectrum	17, 20
benzyl isocyanide	92–93/11	—	2146	U.v. spectrum	17, 20, 22
	48–49/0.5				
styryl isocyanide	—	55–56/0.05	—	Red	105, 106, 107
p-methoxyphenacyl isocyanide	110–111	—	2140	—	106
3-α-colestanyl isocyanide	141–143	—	—	$[\alpha]_D^{16}$ 27° (Ch., *c*, 1.6)	15

[a] all the u.v. spectra are reported in ref. 20; those of phenyl and *p*-tolyl isocyanide also in 37.

Table 1.4 Diisocyanides

Compound	M.p.	B.p.	ν(CN)	Note	Ref.
CN—CH₂—NC	—	—	—	Only in solution	107, 108
CN—(CH₂)₂—NC	—	65–68/0·05 80–81/3	2155	—	17, 111
CN—(CH₂)₄—NC	—	70–75/0·01	2141	—	17, 111
CN—(CH₂)₆NC	—	79–80/0·01	2155	—	108, 111
o-phenylendiisocyanide	—	—	—	—	109
m-phenylendiisocyanide	106–107 (dec)	—	2128, 2105	—	17, 108
p-phenylendiisocyanide	100 (dec) 165 (dec)	—	2128, 2105	Dipole moment: 0 Debye[6]	17, 108
1,3-cyclohexylendiisocyanide	106–107	115–116/1·5	2146	No isomer was separated	17, 108
1,4-cyclohexylendiisocyanide	108–109	110–115/0·1	2137	No isomer was separated	17, 108, 110
p-tetrachlorophenylendi-isocyanide	188–189 (dec)	—	—	—	17, 109
1,4-napthalendiisocyanide	110–112	—	—	—	17, 109
1,5-naphthalendiisocyanide	150 (dec)	—	—	—	17, 109, 110
2,7-naphthalendiisocyanide	142–4	—	—	—	17, 109
2,6-naphthalendiisocyanide	>280 (dec)	—	—	—	111
xanthocylline dimethyl ether	110–111	—	—	Antibiotic	107, 111

Table 1.5 $\Delta\nu$ for CN stretching frequencies of free and complexed isocyanides in various solvents[a]

Solvent	p-tolyl isocyanide[c]	t-butyl isocyanide[c]	Co(CO)(NO)(p-tolyl isocyanide)$_2$ $\Delta\nu_1$	Co(CO)(NO)(p-tolyl isocyanide)$_2$ $\Delta\nu_2$	Co(CO)(NO)[(CH$_3$)$_3$ CNC]$_2$ $\Delta\nu_1$	Co(CO)(NO)[(CH$_3$)$_3$ CNC]$_2$ $\Delta\nu_2$
Carbon disulphide[b]	+1·8	+3·1	−1·9	d	−3·4	d
Cyclohexane	0·0	0·0	0·0	0·0	0·0	0
Toluene	−2·5	−1·6	−10·2	−5·1	−9·3	−9·8
Diethyl-ether	−3·2	−1·7	−9·3	−4·2	−7·5	−9·8
Carbon tetrachloride	−3·7	−2·5	−4·2	−1·4	−3·5	−4·5
CH$_2$I$_2$	−3·7	−4·4	−11·3	−5·7	−12·2	−11·7
Dioxane	−4·5	−3·4	−12·7	−6·6	−12·5	−11·9
2-Butanone	−4·7	−3·4	−15·9	−8·7	−15·2	−13·6
Acetone	−5·0	−4·4	−17·6	−10·2	−16·7	−13·4
CH$_2$Br$_2$	−6·6	−6·0	−13·9	−7·2	−15·3	−15·1
Acetonitrile	−8·4	−6·5	−21·3	−12·0	−21·4	−18·9
Bromoform	−8·4	−8·1	−11·2	−5·6	−12·8	−13·3
Methylene chloride	−8·9	−7·4	−17·6	−10·1	−18·0	−16·2
Chloroform	−9·7	−10·1	−12·7	−7·9	−14·8	−14·0
Vapour phase	−5·0	−2·7	e	e	e	e

[a] All data from ref. 67.
[b] This solvent was found to react very quickly with CH$_3$NC and at various rates with other isocyanides[69].
[c] ν(CN):2120·0, 2131·3, for the isocyanides; 2085·9, 2135·4 and 2108·4, 2141·8 for the two cobalt complexes, respectively.
[d] Obscured by solvent.
[e] Not observable.

Table 1.6 ^1H Chemical shifts and ^1H–^{14}N coupling constant of isocyanides

Compound (neat liquid)	Ref.	Signal			Coupling constant, cps.
		Protons	τ	Multiplicity	
CH_3NC	53	CH_3	7·27	Symm., triplet	$J(N-H):2·4$
CH_3NC (CCl_4)	77	CH_3	7·15	Triplet	$J(N-H):2·7$
C_2H_5—NC	53	CH_2	6·61	Tripled quartet	$J(N-H):2·0$
		CH_3	8·72	Tripled triplet	$J(N-H):2·4$
					$J(H-H):7·3$
$(CH_3)_2CHNC$	53	CH_3	8·55	Tripled doublet	$J(N-H):2·6$
		CH	6·13	Tripled septet	$J(N-H):1·8$
					$J(H-H):7·0$
$CH_3(CH_2)_3NC$	53	α-CH_2	6·70	Tripled triplet shows	$J(N-H):2·0$
		β-CH_2		splitting	$J(H-H):6·7$
$CH_3CH_2CH(CH_3)NC$	53	CH	6·76	Multiplet	$J(CH-CH_3):6·7$
		CH_2	8·38	Multiplet	
		γ-CH_3	8·90	Multiplet	$J(N-CH_3\gamma):2·2$
		CH_3	8·66	Tripled doublet	
$(CH_3)_3CNC$	53	CH_3	8·83	Triplet	$J(N-H):2·4$
$(CH_3)_3CNC$ (CCl_4)	77	CH_3	8·56	Triplet	$J(N-H):3·5$
$C_6H_5CH_2NC$	78	CH_2	5·72	Triplet	$J(N-H):2·7$
$C_6H_{11}NC$	53	CH_2	6·42	Broad	—

Table 1.7 ^{14}N Chemical shifts of isocyanides and nitriles[81]

Compound	Chemical shift[a]	Condition
CH_3NC	240 ± 2	liquid
p-ClC_6H_4NC	201 ± 5	EtOH/MeOH
$1,4$-C_6H_4NC	200 ± 5	EtOH/MeOH
CH_3CN	135 ± 2	liquid
C_6H_5CN	119 ± 3	liquid

[a] In p.p.m. against ammonium nitrate solution as reference.

REFERENCES

1. J. V. Nef, *Annalen*, **270**, 267 (1892).
2. J. V. Nef, *Annalen*, **287**, 265 (1895).
3. I. Langmuir, *J. Am. Chem. Soc.*, **41**, 1543 (1919).
4. H. Lindemann and L. Wiegrebe, *Chem. Ber.*, **63**, 1650 (1930).
5. D. L. Hammick, R. G. A. New, N. V. Sidgwick and L. E. Sutton, *J. Chem. Soc.*, **1930**, 1876.
6. R. G. A. New and L. Sutton, *J. Chem. Soc.*, **1932**, 1415.
7. W. Gordy and L. Pauling, *J. Am. Chem. Soc.*, **64**, 2953 (1942).
8. L. Pauling, *The Nature of Chemical Bond*, Cornell University Press, New York, 1960, pp. 269, 338.
9. C. C. Costain, *J. Chem. Phys.*, **29**, 864 (1958).
10. R. B. King. *Inorg. Chem.*, **6**, 25 (1967); J. F. Guttenberger, *Abstracts*, 3rd International Symposium on Organometallic Chemistry, Munich (1967), p. 96.

11. M. Gautier, *Ann. Chim. et Phys.*, [IV] **17**, 203 (1869).
12. M. Gautier, *Ann. Chim. et Phys.*, [IV] **17**, 222 (1869).
13. W. A. Hofmann, *Ann. Chim. et Phys.*, [IV] **17**, 210 (1869).
14. W. A. Hofmann, *Annalen*, **144**, 117 (1867).
15. W. R. Hertler and E. J. Corey, *J. Org. Chem.*, **23**, 1221 (1958).
16. I. Ugi and R. Meyr, *Angew Chem.*, **70**, 702 (1958).
17. I. Ugi, W. Betz, U. Fetzer and K. Offermann, *Chem. Ber.*, **94**, 2814 (1961);
    I. Ugi, U. Fetzer, E. Eholzer, H. Knupfer and K. Offermann, *Angew. Chem.*, **77**, 492 (1965); *Angew. Chem. (Int. Edit.)*, **4**, 472 (1965).
18. I. Ugi, R. Meyr, M. Lipinski, F. Bodesheim and F. Rosendahl, *Org. Synth.*, **41**, 3 (1961).
19. I. Ugi and R. Meyr, *Org. Synth.*, **41**, 101 (1964).
20. I. Ugi and R. Meyr, *Chem. Ber.*, **93**, 239 (1960).
21. R. Wittmann, *Angew Chem.*, **73**, 219 (1961).
22. *German Patent*, 1,084,715; *Chem. Abstr.*, **55**, 21051i (1961).
23. *Dutch Patent Application*, 6,410,212; *Chem. Abstr.*, **63**, 8272c (1966).
24. *German Patent*, 1,158,499; *Chem. Abstr.*, **60**, 5638a (1963).
25. H. L. Jackson and R. C. McKusick, *Org. Synth.*, Coll. Vol. IV, 438.
26. E. A. V. Ebsworth and S. G. Frankiss, *J. Chem. Soc.*, **1963**, 661.
27. L. Malatesta, *Gazz. Chim. It.*, **77**, 238 (1947).
28. P. A. S. Smith and N. Kalenda, *J. Org. Chem.*, **23**, 1599 (1958).
29. D. Samuel, B. Weinraub and B. Ginsburg, *J. Org. Chem.*, **21**, 376 (1956).
30. H. Feuer, H. Rubinstein and A. T. Nielsen, *J. Org. Chem.*, **23**, 1107 (1958).
31. C. Grundmann, *Chem. Ber.*, **91**, 1380 (1958).
32. A. Sacco, *Gazz. Chim. It.*, **85**, 989 (1955).
33. A. P. Krapcho, *J. Org. Chem.*, **27**, 1089 (1962).
34. T. Shingaki and M. Takebayashi, *Bull. Chem. Soc. Japan*, **36**, 617 (1963).
35. B. V. Tronov and M. I. Bardamova, *Isvest. Visoshikh. Ucheb. Zavednii Khim. i Khim. Tekhnol.* 2, No. 1, 34 (1959); *Chem. Abstr.*, **53**, 21823b (1959).
36. *German Patent*, 1,158,501; *Chem. Abstr.*, **60**, 6795e (1963).
37. T. Mukayama, H. Nambu and M. Okamoto, *J. Org. Chem.*, **27**, 3615 (1962).
38. T. Mukayama and Y. Yokota, *Bull. Chem. Soc. Japan*, **38**, 858 (1965).
39. T. A. Manuel, *Inorg. Chem.*, **3**, 1703 (1964).
40. W. A. Hofmann, *Chem. Ber.*, **3**, 766 (1870).
41. W. Weith, *Chem. Ber.*, **6**, 210 (1873).
42. D. H. Lorenz and E. I. Becker, *J. Org. Chem.*, **28**, 1707 (1963).
43. I. Ugi and K. Rosendahl, unpublished results, mentioned in ref. 176.
44. U. Schmidt and K. A. Kabitze, *Angew. Chem.*, **76**, 687 (1964); *Angew. Chem. (Int. Edit.)*, **3**, 641 (1964).
45. T. Mukayama, K. Tonooka and K. Inoue, *J. Org. Chem.*, **26**, 2202 (1961).
46. T. Mukayama and T. Hata, *Bull. Chem. Soc. Japan*, **33**, 1382 (1960).
47. E. Mueller and B. Narr, *Z. Naturforschung*, **16b**, 845 (1961).
48. W. Z. Heldt, *Adv. Chem. Ser.*, **37**, 99 (1963) and references therein.
49. G. Calmels, *Compt. Rend.*, **98**, 538 (1883).
50. M. Freund, *Chem. Ber.*, **21**, 937 (1888).
51. C. D. Russel and L. Pauling, *Proc. Natl. Acad. Sci. U.S.*, **25**, 517 (1939); R. St. George and L. Pauling, *Science*, **114**, 629 (1951).
52. Toxicologic Laboratory of Farbenfabriken Bayer, mentioned in ref. 17 b.

53. J. Casanova, Jr., N. D. Werner and R. E. Schuster, *J. Org. Chem.*, **31**, 3473 (1966).
54. A. Lifshitz, H. F. Carroll and S. H. Bauer, *J. Am. Chem. Soc.*, **86**, 1448 (1964).
55. F. W. Schneider and B. S. Rabinovitch, *J. Am. Chem. Soc.*, **86**, 2356 (1963).
56. S. Herzog and H. Gutsche, *Z. Chem.*, **3**, 393, (1963).
57. C. E. Coffey, *J. Inorg. Nucl. Chem.*, **25**, 179 (1963).
58. T. Mukayama, M. Tozikawa and N. Takei, *J. Org. Chem.*, **27**, 803 (1962).
59. G. Kohlmaier and B. S. Rabinovitch, *J. Phys. Chem.*, **63**, 1793 (1959).
60. R. W. Horobin, N. R. Khan and J. McKenna, *Tetrahedron Letters*, **1966**, 5087.
61. D. H. Shaw and H. O. Pritchard, *J. Phys. Chem.*, **70**, 1230 (1966).
62. W. Drenth, *Rec. Trav. Chim.*, **81**, 319 (1962).
63. T. Saegusa, Y. Ito, S. Kobayashi and K. Hirota, *Tetrahedron Letters*, **1967**, 521.
64. Y. Yamamoto and N. Hagihara, *Bull. Chem. Soc. Japan*, **39**, 1084 (1966).
65. D. S. Matteson and R. A. Bailey, *Chem. and Ind.*, **1967**, 191.
66. K. Sjoeberg, *Svensk Kemisk Tidskrift*, **75**, 43 (1963).
67. W. D. Horrocks, Jr. and R. H. Mann, *Spectrochim. Acta*, **19**, 1375 (1963).
68. R. G. Gillis and J. L. Occolowitz, *Spectrochim. Acta*, **19**, 873 (1963).
69. F. A. Cotton and F. A. Zingales, *J. Am. Chem. Soc.*, **83**, 351 (1961).
70. T. L. Brown, *J. Am. Chem. Soc.*, **80**, 794 (1958).
71. P. Sensi and G. G. Gallo, *Gazz. Chim. It.*, **85**, 224 (1955).
72. G. C. Pimentel and A. L. McClellan, *The Hydrogen Bond*, W. H. Freeman, S. Francisco and London, 1960, Chap. 3.
73. L. L. Ferstandig, *J. Am. Chem. Soc.*, **84**, 3553 (1962).
74. L. L. Ferstandig, *J. Am. Chem. Soc.*, **84**, 1323 (1962).
75. A. Allerhand and P. Von R. Schleyer, *J. Am. Chem. Soc.*, **85**, 866 (1963).
76. P. von R. Schleyer and A. Allerhand, *J. Am. Chem. Soc.*, **84**, 1322 (1962).
77. I. D. Kuntz, Jr., P. von R. Schleyer and A. Allerhand, *J. Chem. Phys.*, **35**, 1533 (1961).
78. W. Z. Heldt, *Inorg. Chem.*, **2**, 1048 (1963).
79. J. P. Maher, *J. Chem. Soc.*, Part A, **1966**, 1855.
80. J. Casanova, Jr. and R. E. Schuster, *Tetrahedron Letters*, **1964**, 405; J. Casanova, Jr., H. R. Kiefer, D. Kuwada and A. M. Boulton, *Tetrahedron Letters*, 1965, 703.
81. D. Herbison-Evans, and R. E. Richard, *Mol. Phys.*, **8**, 19 (1964).
82. R. G. Gillis and J. L. Occolowitz, *J. Org. Chem.*, **28**, 2924 (1963).
83. J. Casanova, Jr., R. E. Schuster and N. D. Werner, *J. Chem. Soc.*, **1963**, 4280.
84. A. G. Kelso and A. B. Lacey, *J. Chromatog.*, **18**, 156 (1965).
85. R. G. Gillis, *J. Org. Chem.*, **27**, 4103 (1962).
86. M. G. Voronkov, *Latvijas PSR Zinatnu Akad. Vestis. kim. Ser.*, 1961, 25; *Chem. Abstr.*, **57**, 9324c (1963).
87. J. Petruska, *J. Chem. Phys.*, **34**, 1120 (1961).
88. D. E. Milligan, *J. Chem. Phys.*, **39**, 712 (1963).
89. A. G. Allen, E. D. Tidwell and E. K. Plyler, *J. Chem. Phys.*, **25**, 302 (1956).
90. H. Siebert, *Anwendungen der Schwingungsspektroskopie in der anorganischen Chemie*, Springer Verlag, 1966, p. 47.
91. D. H. Rank, G. Shorinko, D. P. Eastman and T. A. Wiggins, *J. Opt. Soc. Amer.*, **50**, 421 (1960).

92. R. H. Williams, *J. Phys. Chem.*, **25**, 656 (1956).
93. S. L. N. G. Krishnamachari, *Indian J. Phys.*, **28**, 463 (1954).
94. M. Bigorgne and A. Bouquet, *J. Organomet. Chem.*, **1**, 101 (1963).
95. F. Cappellina and V. Lorenzelli, *Ann. Chim. (Italy)*, **48**, 855 (1958).
96. S. Otsuka, K. Mori and K. Yamagami, *J. Org. Chem.*, **31**, 4170 (1966).
97. *German Patent*, 1,177,146; *Chem. Abstr.*, **61**, 14536e (1964).
98. I. Ugi and K. Rosendahl, *Annalen*, **666**, 65 (1963).
99. M. Bredereck, B. Foelisch and K. Walz, *Angew. Chem.*, **74**, 388 (1962); *Angew. Chem. (Int. Edit.)*, **1**, 334 (1962).
100. *French Patent*, 1,379,916; *Chem. Abstr.*, **62**, 10370c (1965).
101. A. A. R. Sayigh and H. Ulrich, *J. Chem. Soc.*, **1963**, 3146.
102. S. Bose, *J. Indian Chem. Soc.*, **35**, 376 (1958); *Chem. Abstr.*, **58**, 1033g (1959); *Chem. Zentr.*, **131**, 12640 (1960).
103. T. E. Stevens, *J. Org. Chem.*, **28**, 2436 (1963).
104. *French Patent*, 1,379,917; *Chem. Abstr.*, **62**, 11744c (1965).
105. *German Patent*, 1,168,895; *Chem. Abstr.*, **61**, 4279f (1964).
106. I. Hagedorn and H. Etling, *Angew. Chem.*, **73**, 26 (1961).
107. I. Hagedorn, V. Eholzer and R. Etling, *Chem. Ber.*, **98**, 193 (1965).
108. R. Neidlein, *Angew. Chem.*, **76**, 440 (1964); *Angew. Chem. (Int. Edit.)*, **3**, 382 (1964); R. Neidlein, *Arch. Pharm.*, **297**, 589 (1964).
109. *German Patent*, 1,158,500; *Chem. Abstr.*, **61**, 8243a (1964).
110. *German Patent*, 1,167,332; *Chem. Abstr.*, **61**, 614a (1964).
111. *French Patent*, 1,384,210; *Chem. Abstr.*, **62**, 10384f (1965).
112. R. E. Schuster, J. E. Scott and J. Casanova, Jr., *Org. Synth.*, **46**, 75 (1966).

2 GENERAL PROPERTIES OF ISOCYANIDE COMPLEXES

GENERALITIES

The evidence derived from the studies[1,2,3] on the hydrogen bonding
of isocyanides showed that these can be considered as Lewis bases,
because of the presence of a lone electron pair on the carbon atom.
It is this same electron pair that enables isocyanides to act as ligands
in coordination compounds. Several addition compounds of isocyanides were already known long before the modern theory on the
coordinate bond had been developed, and even before Werner's
general theory on coordination. Organic chemists first came across
these addition compounds while studying the synthesis of alkyl
isocyanides; in fact, the product of the reaction between silver
cyanide and alkylating reagents is an adduct of the type $RNC.AgCN$.

22

In a similar way the esters of 'ferrocyanic acid', which later were recognized to be addition products of iron (II) and alkyl isocyanides, were at first investigated by the organic chemists and considered to be the trialkyl derivatives of the tricyanogen $(R_3C_3N_3)_3Fe$.

It was not unnatural that the acknowledged tendency of alkyl isocyanides to give addition compounds with silver, copper and iron salts led the chemists of that time to extend the research to most of the other metals, and from alkyl to aryl isocyanides. Before 1947, the addition compounds between isocyanides and the following metals were known: Cr^{III}, Fe^{II}, Fe^{III}, Co^{III}, Cu^{I}, Zn^{II}, Mo^{IV}, Ag^{I}, Cd^{II}, Pt^{II}, W^{IV} and Hg^{II}. Some of these compounds, e.g. the derivatives of Fe^{II} and Pt^{II}, had some interest because of their remarkable stability and their occurrence in stereoisomeric forms, but on the whole they did not show any properties to suggest that isocyanides could play a role essentially different from that of the other known ligands.

Today isocyanide complexes are known for many transition elements (from Group VI to Group VIII, Tc and Os excepted), for some post-transition elements (Group I and II) and a few typical elements, such as boron, aluminium and the lanthanides.

The similarity of transition-metal isocyanide complexes to the metal carbonyls was realized rather early, and was nationalized later, mainly on infrared and x-ray structural evidence. The main difference between CO and isocyanide ligands is the value of the dipole moment, which is 0·1 Debye in the former and $\sim 3\cdot4$ Debye for the latter.

An important consequence of the existence of a dipole moment with the negative charge on the terminal carbon of the isocyanides is the remarkable tendency of these ligands to give cationic species, as FeL_6^{2+} or CoL_5^{+}, while no anion containing only isocyanide is known.

The reaction[4]

$$Co_2(CO)_8 + 5\,L \rightarrow [L_5Co][Co(CO)_4] + 4\,CO$$

is illustrative of the difference between CO, which tends to stabilize low oxidation states and anions, and isocyanide (L), which is able to stabilize higher oxidation states and cations.

GENERAL METHODS FOR THE PREPARATION OF ISOCYANIDE COMPLEXES

The most obvious method involves the simple mixing of the metal derivative in the required oxidation state with the ligand, which is often liquid. The method has proved itself useful in all those reactions, such as Fe^{II} [5], where the product is rather robust and polymerization is not catalysed by the metal compound employed, as it is, for example, by nickel (II) salts[6]. The use of a solvent, to moderate the reaction, is imperative in some cases: the heat of the reaction may bring about some reduction of the complex, as it does with rhenium (III) complexes[7]. Often a complex in a higher oxidation state, e.g. Co^{II}, is reduced by the excess ligand to a lower oxidation state simply by boiling[8]. Sometimes an excess of ligand is absolutely necessary as illustrated by Cr^{II} conversion to Cr^0 isocyanide derivatives[9]; in other cases, e.g. Mo, a well-defined set of reaction conditions and a reducing agent is required and, even so, bad yields of Mo^0 (or W^0) compounds are obtained[10].

Another method comprises the displacement of a different ligand. Partial displacement of carbon monoxide is generally possible, but the displacement may not go further than two carbonyls as in iron pentacarbonyl. Total displacement of carbon monoxide is generally very difficult, although possible in $C_5H_5Fe(CO)_2 I$ [11]. The preparative value is slight, since the drastic reaction conditions necessary for the substitution facilitate the formation of polymers from the unreacted ligand. In some other cases, a compound like $Mo(CO)_4$-$(CNR)_2$ can be obtained directly from the carbonyl by refluxing in an inert solvent until the required quantity of carbon monoxide is evolved; but the reaction product may have a tendency to disproportionate[12]:

$$2 \ Mo(CO)_4L_2 \rightleftarrows Mo(CO)_5L + Mo(CO)_3L_3$$

and all the possible products are then present in the reaction mixture. Therefore, cycloheptatriene[13], cyclooctadiene or ammonia[14] derivatives of metal carbonyls are prepared as intermediates and these are then reacted with isocyanide. In a few cases, the displaced ligand has been a halide ion[12], dipyridyl[15] or ethanol[16].

The third method is the alkylation of alkali or silver cyanometallates with active alkyl or aryl halides[17], alkyl sulphate[18] and even organometallic halides[19]. The method often requires long reaction times. Sometimes rather complicated mixtures have been obtained and some of the published results look suspicious, especially those in the older literature.

The last method involves reaction of an isocyanate or isothiocyanate with a metal carbonyl, according to the equation:

$$M(CO)_n + RNCO \rightarrow (RNC)M(CO)_{n-1} + CO_2$$

This method was discovered quite recently[20] and as yet little is known about its general validity.

Thin-layer chromatography can be very useful for purification of isocyanide complexes and for ascertaining their purity. Since there has been no discussion of this in the published literature, some details[21] are given here, the successful separation of $M(CO)_{6-n}$-$(CNPh)_n$ (M = Cr,Mo,W; n = 1, 2, 3) serving as an example. Silica gel G was used. A small quantity of a polar solvent (5%) in a non-polar one afforded adequate separation. In the absence of the polar solvent there was no separation, while an excess gave tailing and did not afford a good separation of the compound either. The conditions used are reported in detail in Table. 2.1.

THE EFFECT OF COORDINATION ON THE INFRARED SPECTRA OF ISOCYANIDES

Terminal isocyanide groups

When an isocyanide molecule coordinates to a metal ion, there is generally a change in the infrared spectrum. The most important change is the shifting of the CN stretching frequency. The quantitative value of the shift (up or down) is generally much more than the rise of a few cm^{-1} resulting from a pure kinematic coupling.

When an isocyanide coordinates to a typical element, such as boron or aluminium, or to a mono- or di-positive cation, there is a rise in the CN stretching frequency which may be up to or even in excess of $100\ cm^{-1}$. The increase of the frequency indicates a higher bond order in the complex than in the free ligand. In the language of the valence-bond theory, it is said that the weight of the canonical structure **2** is higher than that of structure **1**, where α has to be $< 180°$.

$$R \diagdown \underset{N}{\overset{\alpha}{\diagup}} = C = M \qquad\qquad R-N \equiv C \rightarrow M$$

$$(\mathbf{1})\ \ (\alpha < 180°) \qquad\qquad\qquad (\mathbf{2})$$

In the language of the molecular-orbital theory, it is said that there is no significant electron flow towards the π^* orbitals of the ligand. The type of bonding is comparable to that present in ether or amine complexes[22], i.e. the isocyanide functions as a pure donor ligand.

When an isocyanide coordinates to a transition element in a low oxidation state, e.g. zerovalent nickel or chromium, the value of

2+I.C.M.

the $\nu(\text{CN})$ is lower in the complex than in the free ligand. The lowering of the bond order is attributed to a substantial contribution of structure **1** or a substantial electron flow from the metal d orbitals to the antibonding π orbitals on the ligand. This is quite analogous to the behaviour of other π-bonding ligands, such as carbon monoxide or PF_3 [23].

It is one of the remarkable properties of isocyanides, however, that they may behave either as good π-acceptors or as good σ-donors, as evidenced, *inter alia*, by the formation of complexes with trialkylboron and with zerovalent transition elements. Few other ligands complex effectively with *both* of these kinds of acceptors.

A semi-quantitative expression of these underlying concepts and an infrared criterion for measuring the π-bonding ability of isocyanides as ligands, was first found by Cotton[23]. The infrared spectrum of various $M(\text{CNR})_6^{n+}$ compounds ($M = \text{Cr}$, Mo, $n = 0$; $M = \text{Mn}$, $n = 1, 2$) were recorded in the $\nu(\text{CN})$ region[24]. It was realized that zerovalent compounds showed remarkable (60–200 cm^{-1}) decreases in $\nu(\text{CN})$; decreases, but to a lesser extent (12–40 cm^{-1}), were present in Mn^{I} compounds; an increase ($\sim 30 \text{ cm}^{-1}$) was observed in the similar Mn^{II} compounds. In the last case, the importance of the polar structure **2** will be enhanced by the presence of positive formal charge on the cation; as a consequence, there will be a rather high bond order, and the observed rise in $\nu(\text{CN})$. A similar effect explains the rise of $\nu(\text{CN})$ in Mn^{I} derivatives; the numerical value of $\varDelta\nu$ is lower than that of Mn^{II} derivatives, owing to the smaller formal charge. No such mechanism will be operative in zerovalent compounds; instead, owing to the principle of electroneutrality, there is a tendency to disperse the charge accumulated on the metal atom by back-donation to the ligands. Therefore structure **1** will be favoured, with a consequent lowering of the bond order and the observed decrease in the CN stretching frequency. The lowering of the CN stretching frequency will be roughly proportional to the amount of back-donation (or double bonding) for the ligand.

Investigation of two related compounds, $L_2\text{Ag}^+$ ($\nu(\text{CN}):2195$) and $L_4\text{Ag}^+$($\nu(\text{CN}):2177$), ($L = p$-tolylisocyanide, $\nu(\text{CN}):2136$), gave additional support to the idea that back-donation is larger in complexes with a higher negative charge, here carried over by the third and fourth ligand. The influence of the nature of R in CNR on the infrared CN stretching frequency of complexes with π-bonding was also investigated by Cotton[24]. He found that methylisocyanide is a poorer π-acceptor than arylisocyanides; the result was later confirmed by Bigorgne, who examined the 'courbes de filiation' for $Mo(CO)_{6-n}(CNR)_n$ ($n = 1, 2, 3$)[25]. Further, there was no remarkable difference in the CN stretching frequency for the complexes examined by Cotton when the *para* substituent in the arylisocyanide varied from H to CH_3, CH_3O and Cl.

Comparison of isocyanide with other ligands

The infrared criterion allowed a classification of various π-accepting ligands by synthesizing suitable $M(CO)_xL_y$ compounds and comparing their CO and, in the present case, CN stretching frequencies. While isocyanide ligands alone seem to be able to allow back-donation as extensive as carbon monoxide does, the situation is different when both carbon monoxide and isocyanide are bonded to the same metal atom. When only one isocyanide ligand is present, e.g. $(CNR)Mo(CO)_5$, the infrared criterion suggests that back-bonding is virtually all towards the five carbonyl groups. When more than one isocyanide group is present, they accept some back-donation, but this is always lower than where isocyanides are the only ligands. The π-accepting ability of isocyanides in carbonyl complexes is therefore lower than that of CO and is generally considered to be slightly better than that of triarylphosphines.

According to the spectral work by Horrocks[26] a sort of 'spectrochemical series' for π-bonding ligands can be arranged, as follows:

NO	$PCl_2(OC_2H_5)$	$PCl(Oc_6H_5)_2$	$S(C_2H_5)_2$
CO	$PCl_2C_6H_5$	p-tolylisocyanide	$As(C_2H_5)_3$
PF_3	PBr_2CH_3	$P(OCH_3)_3$	$P(CH_3)_3$
$SbCl_3$	$As(OCH_3)_3$	t-butylisocyanide	$P(C_2H_5)_3$
$AsCl_3$	$PCl(OC_4H_9)_2$	$As(NC_5H_{10})_3$	o-$C_6H_4[P(C_2H_5)_2]_2$
PCl_3	$As(OC_2H_5)_3$	$As(C_6H_5)_3$	o-phenantroline
$PCl_2(OC_4H_9)$	$P(OC_6H_5)_3$	$P(C_6H_5)_3$	diethylenetriamine

The arrangement is in order of decreasing ability to withdraw charges from the central metal atom, by either an inductive or π-electron mechanism.

Similar results were obtained by examination of a suitably substituted series of $M(CO)_5L$ compounds (M = Cr, Mo). The same conclusion was reached by considering either the $v(CO)$, the approximate force constants[27] (Table 2.2) or the 'rigorous' force constants[28]. On similar and different[28a] compounds the same conclusion was also reached by Bigorgne[25], through the 'courbes de filiation' of

$Mo(CO)_{6-n}(RNC)_n$ ($n = 1, 2, 3$) compounds (Figures 4.2, 4.3). Strohmeier obtained the same results on a rather different type of compound, (aromatic)$Cr(CO)_2(L)$, using a sensitive method of determination[29]. The same author also found that isocyanides have better π-accepting abilities than nitriles (p. 60). These last results will be discussed in Chapter 4 under chromium.

Solvent effect

Although the solvent effect observed on the $\nu(CN)$ of the isocyanides ought not to be present in coordinated isocyanides, since the interested bond is embedded in a molecule and not free to interact with the solvent, the reverse is true, as can be seen from Table 1.5, which gives the actual values of $\Delta\nu$ (up to 10 cm^{-1}). There are several factors which may contribute to the observed differences and a discussion of them can be found in the literature[30]. All this stresses the need to apply the infrared criterion for evaluating the π-accepting ability of a series of ligands using measurements in the same solvent, as done for the 'spectrochemical series' reported before.

From the frequent appearance in the $\nu(CN)$ region of more bands than those required by simple application of group theory, it was often concluded that the M—C—N—R grouping does not lie on a straight line. The distortion was generally ascribed to steric hindrance of the isocyanide group or to a small contribution of structure 1, which is not linear. Small deviations of the C—N—R angle from 180° were indeed reported in some complexes[31,32,33,34]. Further, a decidedly non-linear CNR moiety was found in a molecule containing bridging isocyanide[35]. In any event, care should be taken when recording spectra in chlorinated hydrocarbons, since evidence for partial decomposition of some complex is now available[36].

Bridging isocyanide groups

Bridging isocyanide groups are not common. Three complexes with a CNR group bridging between two metal atoms have been characterized, namely $[C_5H_5Ni(CNC_6H_5)]_2$[35,37], $[C_5H_5Ni(CNC_6H_{11})]_2$[6] and $(C_5H_5)_2Fe_2(CO)_3(CNC_6H_5)$[35], and one more is reported, $[(C_5H_5Fe(CO)(CNC_6H_5)]_2$[35]. In these compounds the CN stretching frequency is much lower than usual (around 1700 cm^{-1}), as in the case of the bridging compared with the terminal carbonyl groups[38]. The remarkably low bond order for the CN bond enhances the contribution of structure **1** to give in the crystal a C—N—Ar angle of $131°$ [35].

A low value of the CN stretching frequency (1757 cm^{-1}) was found in the yellow form of $[Pd(CNC_6H_{11})_2]_n$ [39] and a novel form of coordinated isocyanide was proposed:

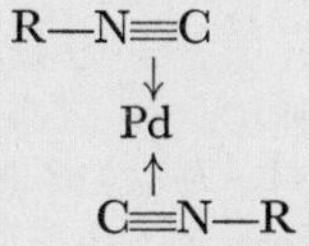

$$
\begin{array}{c}
R—N\equiv C \\
\downarrow \\
Pd \\
\uparrow \\
C\equiv N—R
\end{array}
$$

There is no reason for discarding *a priori* such a suggestion, especially in view of the fact that a similar mode of bonding is known for succinonitrile complexes[40]. However, comparison of the value reported[39] and those of bridging isocyanides would not exclude a structure like

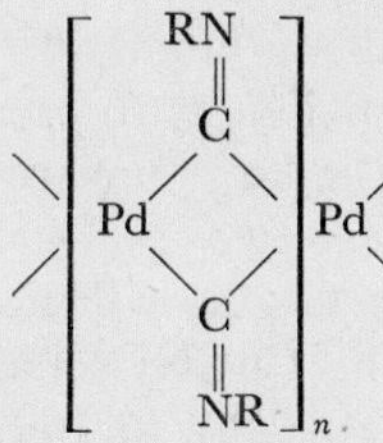

$$
\left[
\begin{array}{c}
RN \\
\parallel \\
C \\
\diagup \diagdown \\
\diagdown Pd \diagdown \quad \diagup Pd \diagup \\
\diagup \quad \diagdown \diagup \quad \diagdown \\
C \\
\parallel \\
NR
\end{array}
\right]_n
$$

as suggested by Malatesta[41].

The possibility of isolating two isomers where the same unchanged ligand has two different ways of attachment to the metal is a limiting case. The equilibrium between two forms, like $[C_5H_5Ni(CNC_6H_{11})]$ with or without bridging isocyanide[6], must be considered as an intermediate case; this type of equilibrium is already well stabilized in the case of bridging carbonyls[42]. No similar study is available for an isocyanide complex.

X-RAY STRUCTURAL DATA

Some x-ray structural determinations have been carried out up to now on certain methyl isocyanide complexes of iron, copper and cobalt and on one phenyl isocyanide complex where the ligand is bridging between two iron atoms. The relevant data are reported in Table 2.2.

It is evident that the M—C—N grouping is practically linear in all the terminal isocyanide complexes investigated so far; small differences from 180° were found, but their reality is not certain. Also, the C—N—C group was found to be practically linear in terminal isocyanide complexes. The value of 167° reported for *trans*-Fe-$(CNCH_3)_4(CN)_2$ cannot be considered, since the work is of 'low accuracy by present standards'[32]. Similarly, the standard deviations are sufficiently large that the variances from 180° for $[Co_2(CNCH_3)_{10}]^{4+}$ may not be significant.

The C—NCH_3 bond length is 1.14 ± 0.02 Å in the two cobalt complexes, and is reported to be around 1.2 Å in the other complexes. The values are not very different from the value of the same bond length in methylisocyanide (1.166 Å). Although lengthening of the bond on coordination is expected, the increase cannot be much, owing to the apparent insensitivity of some bond lengths when the bond order is higher than 2. For example, the terminal CO bond length in carbonyl molecules are always around 1.16 Å, not much higher than the length in carbon monoxide (1.13 Å).

The N—CH_3 bond length is not different from the value found in the free ligand (1.42), if the large uncertainty involved in some of the reported values is considered.

The determination of the C—N—CH_3 angle in the cobalt complexes gave evidence that the CoCNC chain is linear. Comparison of the value reported in Table 2.2 for terminal isocyanides shows that the angle deviates very little from 180° (less than 10°) in all cases. This happens in complexes where little back-donation is present, as in iron (II) derivatives, according to infrared evidence. The value of the CNC angle is then in agreement with a high contribution of structure **2** (p. 25); or, in the MO language, that there is a very small back flow of d_π electrons into π-antibonding CN orbitals.

The CNC angle is not very different from 180° where there is appreciable back-donation, as evidenced from the short Co—C distance $(1.87 \pm 0.015$ Å) in $[Co(CNCH_3)_5]^+$. The single bond Co—C distance is assumed[31] to be 2.15 ± 0.05 Å; and certainly not less than 2.00 Å, even in the most unfavourable case. So, the shortening of the bond is 0.25–0.30 Å and certainly > 0.13 in the most unfavourable case. Evaluation of this decrease in the bond length by comparison with other established examples of back-bonding (e.g. C—Ni in $Ni(CO)_4$ 1.82 Å, against an estimated value of 2.16), brings the conclusion that the Co—C bond order in $[Co(CNCH_3)_5]^+$ is at least 1.5 and, perhaps greater[32]. Such a high contribution of the structure **2** (p. 25), in terms of valence-bond language, would necessarily require a CNC angle sensibly smaller than 180°. The maximum CNC angle compatible with the reported x-ray data can only be 177° − 3 × standard deviation, i.e. 172·5°. Such an angle would then allow only a M—C bond order of 1·17[32] against the value of > 1·5.

The conclusion was therefore reached that the 'valence-bond treatment of the metal isonitrile back-bonding is not satisfactory'[32], at least the simple VB treatment. This conclusion could not have been reached on the basis of the infrared spectra, which can be interpreted by both treatments.

OTHER DATA

All the isocyanide complexes with an even number of d electrons are diamagnetic; those complexes with an odd number of d electrons, such as those of Mn^{II} and Co^{II}, have the low spin configuration, i.e. their effective magnetic moments are $\sim 1·8$ BM[43,44]. In the formally Ni^{I} derivatives, the compounds are diamagnetic owing to a nickel-nickel bond[6]. A metal–metal bond was also invoked[45] to explain the diamagnetism in the solid state of the violet form of $Co(CNR)_4X_2$, which, however, is paramagnetic in chloroform solution. A few e.s.r. data are now available for Co^{II} complexes[65,66].

The paramagnetic nature of Ni^{II} and Co^{II} acetylacetonates was exploited to study their labile 1:1 complex with phenyl and p-tolyl isocyanide by ^1H n.m.r.[46].

The electronic spectra of isocyanide complexes have been recorded in a few cases. They are reported in the table under the appropriate compound; they were employed by Sacco to establish the coordination of some cobalt complexes[43]. No band assignment is reported, with the exception of the work done by Carassiti[47] on $[Fe(CNCH_3)_6]$-Cl_2, during a study on the photochemical decomposition of the complex.

Similarly, very little is known about the polarographic behaviour of isocyanide complexes. $[Fe(CNCH_3)_6]Cl_2$ gave two polarographic waves, the first one being assigned to direct reduction of Fe^{II} to 'metallic iron', while the second one was not definitely assigned[48]. Some additional polarographic work on iron complexes has been reported by Heldt[49], but no definite conclusions were reached.

Kinetic data are available on a few reactions involving isocyanides. The exchange reaction of $Ni(CNPh)_4$ with ^{14}C-phenyl isocyanide was found too fast to be conveniently followed at 4° C. A similar exchange reaction of $Cr(CNPh)_6$ was studied in benzene solution at a different temperature and an S_N1 dissociative mechanism was deduced[50], the rate being lower than when ^{14}CO was exchanged with $Cr(CO)_6$. Rates of reaction of $Mn(CO)_5Br$ with ethyl isocyanide in chlorobenzene were determined by Angelici and Basolo[51]; this reaction manifested specific solvent effects.

Dipole moments have been measured for a few isocyanide complexes and are given in Table 2·3. These data will be discussed under the relevant element, together with the other lines of available evidence.

Solid state conductivity data[52] and Mössbauer spectra[53] are available for some iron compounds; they too will be mentioned later together with the appropriate compounds.

Table 2.1 R_F and conditions for thin-layer chromatographic separation of some isocyanide complexes[21]

$M(CO)_5(CNPh)$	$M(CO)_4(CNPh)_2$	$M(CO)_3(CNPh)_3$	Eluent[a]
	(M = Chromium)		
0·28	—	0·02	n-pentane
0·28	—	not eluted	n-pentane
		0·04	P.ether[b]
		0·11	n-heptane/ether
		0·13	P.ether[b]/acetone
		0·16	n-pentane/acetone
	(M = Molybdenum)		
0·29	0·05	not eluted	n-pentane
0·29	0·06	not eluted	n-heptane
0·39	0·11	0·02	P.ether[b]
0·43	0·18	0·06	n-heptane/ether
0·53	0·25	0·08	P.ether[b]/acetone
0·62	0·30	0·11	n-pentane/acetone
	(M = Tungsten)		
0·30	0·06	—	n-pentane
0·26	0·05	—	n-heptane
0·35	0.08	—	P.ether[b]
0·49	0·23	—	P.ether[b]/acetone
0·50	0·24	—	n-heptane/acetone
0·59	0·27	—	n-pentane/acetone

[a] When two eluents were used, the second was 5%.
[b] P.ether is a commercial petroleum ether having b.p. 30–50°C.

Table 2.2 Structural data on isocyanides and isocyanide complexes

Complex	Ref.	Structure	Ligand Parameter					
			M—C	C—N	CH_3—N	M—C—N angle	C—N—C angle	M—M
$[Fe(CNCH_3)_6]Cl_2 \cdot 3\,H_2O$	34	octahedral	1.85	1.18	1.47	180	173	
$trans$-$Fe(CNCH_3)_4(CN)_2$	55	distorted octahedral	1.8 ± 0.1	1.3	1.4	180	167 ± 5	
$Cu(CNCH_3)I$	54	see figure (p. 39)	1.81 ± 0.02	1.24	1.30	(180)	174	{2.89 3.42
$[Co_2(CNCH_3)_{10}](ClO_4)_4$ (red)	31	idealized D_{4d}	1.82–1.92 ± 0.04	1.15	1.50 ± 0.05	174 ± 3	172 ± 3	2.7
$[Co(CNCH_3)_5](ClO_4)$	32	trigonal bipyramid	1.87 ± 0.015	1.14 ± 0.02	1.44 ± 0.03	180	177 ± 1.5	
$(C_5H_5)_2Fe_2(CO)_3(CNC_6H_5)$	35	see figure (p. 3)	1.90			138	131	2.5
CH_3NC (Electr. diffr.)	56			1.18	1.44			
CH_3NC (Microwave)	{57 58			1.166	1.424		180°	
t-BuNC(Microwave)	59			1.175	1.420		linear	

Table 2.3   Dipole moments of isocyanide complexes

Compound	Debye	Ref.
R—NC	3·5	60
$Fe(CO)_4(CNCH_3)$	5·02 ± 0·04	61
$p\text{-}(CO_2CH_3)_2C_6H_4Cr(CO)_2(CNC_6H_{11})$	4·48	62
$C_5H_5Mn(CO)_2(CNC_6H_{11})$	4·64	62
$Cr(CO)_5(CNC_6H_{11})$	5·62	62
$Cr(CO)_4(CNC_6H_{11})_2$	0	62
$Mo(CO)_5(CNC_6H_{11})$	5·70	62
$Co(NO)(4\text{-}CH_3C_6H_4NC)_3$	5·29	63
$Co(NO)(4\text{-}CH_3OC_6H_4NC)_3$	5·78	63
$Co(NO)(4\text{-}ClC_6H_4NC)_3$	3·33	63
$Pd(CNC_6H_{11})_2$	2·91	38
$PdI_2(CNC_6H_5)_2$	1·53	64
$PdI_2(4\text{-}ClC_6H_4NC)_2$	1·10	64
$PdI_2(4\text{-}CH_3C_6H_4NC)_2$	1·93	64
$PdI_2(4\text{-}CH_3OC_6H_4NC)_2$	2·53	64
$PdBr_2(4\text{-}CH_3OC_6H_4NC)_2$	2·79	64

REFERENCES

1. R. G. Gillis and J. L. Occolowitz, *Spectrochim. Acta*, **19**, 873 (1963).
2. L. L. Ferstanding, *J. Am. Chem. Soc.*, **84**, 3553 (1962).
3. A. Allerhand and P. von Ragué Schleyer, *J. Am. Chem. Soc.*, **85**, 866 (1963).
4. A. Sacco, *Gazz. Chim. Ital.*, **83**, 622 (1953).
5. L. Malatesta, *Gazz. Chim. Ital.*, **77**, 340 (1963).
6. Y. Yamamoto and N. Hagihara, *Bull. Chem. Soc. Japan*, **39**, 1084 (1966).
7. M. Freni and V. Valenti, *Gazz. Chim. Ital.*, **91**, 1352 (1961).
8. L. Malatesta and A. Sacco, *Z. anorg. Chem.*, **273**, 247 (1953); L. Malatesta and A. Sacco, *Atti Accad. naz. Lincei, Rend. Classe Sci. fis. mat. nat.*, VIII, **15**, 94 (1953).
9. L. Malatesta, A. Sacco and S. Ghielmi, *Gazz. Chim. Ital.*, **82**, 516 (1952).
10. L. Malatesta, A. Sacco and M. Gabaglio, *Gazz. Chim. Ital.*, **82**, 548 (1952).
11. K. K. Joshi, P. L. Pauson and W. H. Stubbs, *J. Organomet. Chem.*, **1**, 51 (1963).
12. H. D. Murdock and R. Henzi, *J. Organomet. Chem.*, **5**, 166 (1966).
13. G. Cetini, O. Gambino and M. Castiglioni, *Atti R. Accad. Sci. Torino, Classe Sci. fis. mat.*, **97**, 1131 (1963) and references therein.
14. W. Hieber, W. Abeck and H. K. Platzer, *Z. anorg. Chem.*, **280**, 253 (1955).
15. S. Herzog and E. Gutsche, *Z. Chem.*, **3**, 393 (1963).
16. F. Canziani, U. Sartorelli and F. Cariati, *Ann. Chim. (Italy)*, **54**, 1354 (1964).
17. W. Z. Heldt, *Adv. Chem. Ser.*, **37**, 99 (1963).
18. E. G. J. Hartley, *J. Chem. Soc.*, **97**, 1066 (1910).
19. R. B. King, *Inorg. Chem.*, **6**, 25 (1967).
20. H. Ulrich, B. Tucker and A. A. R. Sayigh, *Tetrahedron Letters*, **1967**, 731.

21. G. Cetini, private communication (Rome, April 1967).

22. F. A. Cotton and G. Wilkinson, *Advanced Inorganic Chemistry*, 1966.

23. F. A. Cotton and R. V. Parish, *J. Chem. Soc.*, **1960**, 1440.

24. F. A. Cotton and F. Zingales, *J. Am. Chem. Soc.*, **83**, 351 (1961).

25. M. Bigorgne and A. Bouquet, *J. Organomet. Chem.*, **1**, 101 (1963).

26. W. D. Horrocks, Jr. and R. Craig Taylor, *Inorg. Chem.*, **2**, 723 (1963).

27. F. A. Cotton, *Inorg. Chem.*, **3**, 703 (1964).

28. G. R. Van Ecke and W. D. Horrocks, Jr., *Inorg. Chem.*, **5**, 1960 (1966).

28a. W. D. Horrocks, Jr. and R. Craig Taylor, *Inorg. Chem.*, **3**, 584 (1965).

29. W. Strohmeier and H. Hellmann, *Chem. Ber.*, **97**, 1877 (1964).

30. W. D. Horrocks, Jr. and R. H. Mann, *Spectrochim. Acta*, **19**, 1375 (1963).

31. F. A. Cotton, T. G. Dunne and J. S. Wood, *Inorg. Chem.*, **3**, 1495 (1964).

32. F. A. Cotton, T. G. Dunne and J. S. Wood, *Inorg. Chem.*, **4**, 318 (1965).

33. H. M. Powell and G. B. Stanger, *J. Chem. Soc.*, **1939**, 1105.

34. H. M. Powell and G. W. R. Bartindale, *J. Chem. Soc.*, **1945**, 799.

35. K. K. Joshi, O. S. Mills, P. L. Pauson, B. W. Shaw and W. H. Stubbs, *Chem. Comm.*, **1965**, 181.

36. C. H. Bamford, G. C. Eastmond and K. Hargreaves, *Nature*, **205**, 385 (1965).

37. P. L. Pauson and W. H. Stubbs, *Angew. Chem.*, **74**, 466 (1962); *Angew. Chem. (Int. Ed.)*, **1**, 333 (1962).

38. E. W. Abel, *Quart. Rev.*, **17**, 133 (1963).

39. E. O. Fischer and H. Werner, *Chem. Ber.*, **95**, 703 (1962).

40. M. F. Farona and N. J. Brenner, *J. Am. Chem. Soc.*, **88**, 3735 (1966).

41. L. Malatesta, R. Ugo and S. Cenini, *Adv. Chem. Ser.*, **62**, 351 (1967).

42. F. A. Cotton and G. Yagupsky, *Inorg. Chem.*, **6**, 15 (1967); R. D. Fischer, A. Vogler and V. Noack, *J. Organomet. Chem.*, **7**, 135 (1967).

43. A. Sacco and F. A. Cotton, *J. Am. Chem. Soc.*, **84**, 2043 (1962).

44. F. A. Cotton and R. H. Holm, *J. Am. Chem. Soc.*, **83**, 2083 (1963).

45. F. Canziani, F. Cariati and U. Sartorelli, *Ist. Lomb. (Rend. Sc.)*, **A98**, 564 (1964).

46. W. D. Horrocks, Jr., R. Craig Taylor and G. N. La Mar, *J. Am. Chem. Soc.*, **86**, 3031 (1964).

47. V. Carassiti, G. Condorelli and L. L. Condorelli-Costanzo, *Ann. Chim. (Italy)*, **55**, 329 (1965).

48. F. Cappellina and V. Lorenzelli, *Ann. Chim. (Italy)*, **48**, 855 (1958).

49. W. Z. Heldt, *Inorg. Chem.*, **2**, 1048 (1963).

50. G. Cetini and O. Gambino, *Ann. Chim. (Italy)*, **52**, 236 (1963).

51. R. G. Angelici and F. Basolo, *J. Am. Chem. Soc.*, **84**, 2495 (1962).

52. W. Z. Heldt and C. D. Weis, *J. Phys. Chem.*, **67**, 1392 (1963).

53. R. R. Berrett and B. W. Fitzsimmons, *J. Chem. Soc., Part A*, **1967**, 525.

54. P. J. Fisher, N. E. Taylor and M. M. Harding, *J. Chem. Soc.*, **1960**, 2303.

55. R. Hulme and H. M. Powell, *J. Chem. Soc.*, **1957**, 719.

56. W. Gordy and L. Pauling, *J. Am. Chem. Soc.*, **64**, 2953 (1942); W. Kessler, H. Ring, R. Trambarulo and W. Gordy, *Phys. Rev.*, **79**, 54 (1950).

57. C. C. Costain, *J. Chem. Phys.*, **29**, 864 (1958).

58. T. S. Jaseja, *Proc. Indian Acad. Sci.*, **50A**, 108 (1959).

59. B. Bak, L. Hansen-Nygard and J. Rastrup-Andersen, *J. Mol. Spectroscopy*, **2**, 54 (1958).

60. R. G. A. New and L. Sutton, *J. Chem. Soc.*, **1932**, 1415.
61. W. Hieber and E. Weiss, *Z. anorg. allg. Chem.*, **287**, 223 (1956).
62. W. Strohmeier and H. Hellmann, *Ber. Bunsenges. Physik. Chem.*, **68**, 481 (1964).
63. L. Malatesta and A. Sacco, *Z. anorg. Chem.*, **273**, 341 (1953).
64. M. Angoletta, *Ann. Chim.* (*Italy*), **45**, 970 (1955).
65. J. P. Maher, *Chem. Comm.*, **1967**, 332.
66. J. M. Pratt and P. R. Silverman, *Chem. Comm.*, **1967**, 117.

3 ISOCYANIDE COMPLEXES OF THE MAIN-GROUP ELEMENTS

ISOCYANIDE COMPOUNDS OF THE ELEMENTS OF GROUPS IB AND IIB

It is well known that the elements of the B group do not form pure metal carbonyls, and that only those of Group IB give carbonyl halides. The tendency of these elements to form compounds with isocyanides is limited. In Group IB the affinity toward isocyanides, generally strong, increases with the atomic number, while in Group IIB it is rather weak and varies irregularly, showing a maximum for cadmium and a minimum for mercury. If, however, the relative instability of mercury derivatives is ascribed to its tendency to be reduced to Hg_2^{2+}, then the same regularity as in Group IB can be observed.

In their isocyanide derivatives the metals of Groups IB and IIB have an electronic structure with 18 external electrons and display the usual oxidation state corresponding to their group. Only gold also forms rather unstable complexes in the trivalent state. Some of these isocyanide complexes were among the first to be prepared. They have since been reinvestigated, but on the whole the available experimental material is still rather incomplete and not organized in a satisfactory scheme.

Some interesting additions of organic compounds with an active hydrogen, such as alcohols or amines, to isocyanide are catalysed by copper (I) salts, probably via an intermediate mixed complex.

Copper

The alkylation of copper (I) cyanide with alkyl iodides was studied by Guillemard (1867)[1] and later by Hartley[2]. The reaction is analogous to that with silver cyanide, but the yield of isocyanides is rather lower. As in the case of silver the reaction takes place in several stages[2].

At a temperature not higher than 100°, and without solvent, the labile adduct 3 $CuCN.CH_3I$ is formed, from which the methyl iodide can be recovered on heating. In the presence of acetonitrile as solvent, or also, but not so neatly, without solvent at 135°, a stable compound is obtained, which can be crystallized from acetonitrile and has a composition corresponding to $CuCN.CH_3I$. As this product gives off isocyanide on treatment either with potassium cyanide or with silver sulphate, it is to be considered the iodo-(methyl isocyanide) copper(I), $CuI(CNCH_3)$:

$$CuI(CNCH_3) + 3\ KCN \rightarrow K_2Cu(CN)_3 + KI + CH_3NC$$
$$CuI(CNCH_3) + Ag_2SO_4 \rightarrow AgI + Ag + CuSO_4 + CH_3NC$$

It was found later that, when the components are heated in a sealed tube, very little of this compound is formed if the duration of heating is less than 12 hours or if the concentration of methyl iodide in the solvent is less than 35% by volume[3]. At a higher temperature, the cyano(methyl isocyanide)copper (I) is formed:

$$CuI(CNCH_3) + CuCN \rightarrow CuCN(CNCH_3) + CuI$$

An x-ray structural determination on $CuI(CNCH_3)$ supports the chemical evidence[4], although it gives no additional evidence that the ligand is methyl isocyanide rather than acetonitrile. The structure is depicted in Figure 3.1. There are double chains of copper and iodine atoms running parallel to the c-axis. One copper atom, at the centre of the chain, is bonded tetrahedrally to four iodine atoms at

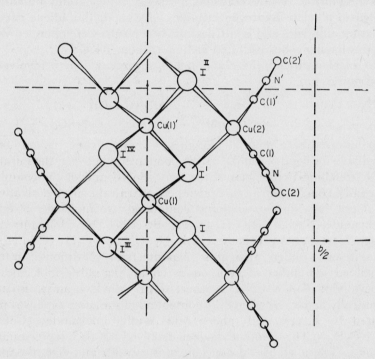

Figure 3.1 Projection of the structure $CuI(CNCH_3)$ along
a-axis

2·64 and 2·67 Angstrom. The other copper atom, on alternate sides of the chain, is bonded tetrahedrally to two iodine atoms, shared with the previously mentioned copper atom, at 2·73 Å and the two CH_3NC groups which are at the side of the chain. The angle CNC in the methylisonitrile group is 174°, 'only possibly significantly different from 180°'. The distance between the two kinds of copper atom (3·42 Å) does not suggest more than a weak bond, while the short distances (2·88 Å) between successive Cu(1) atoms along the chain suggests some kind of interaction.

While generally the reaction of olefins with hydrogen cyanide yields nitriles, the same reaction affords good yields of isonitrile complexes when copper (I) bromide is present. In these reactions, a mixture of bromo(alkyl isocyanide)copper (I) and cyano(alkyl isocyanide)copper (I) is formed, their ratio depending, *inter alia*, upon the solvent. From both complexes aqueous KCN yields free alkyl isonitrile. While ethylene, propene, butenes and butadiene failed to alkylate hydrogen cyanide, 2,3-dimethylbutadiene gave a mixture of nitriles and isonitriles; the best results were obtained with olefins having a disubstituted olefinic carbon, $RRC:$.[5]

A mechanism for the reaction was suggested, which involves a carbonium ion:

$$HCN + CuBr \rightarrow H^+[NC.CuBr]^- \xrightarrow{C_4H_8} t\text{-}Bu^+[NC.CuBr]^- \rightarrow$$
$$t\text{-}BuNC.CuBr \xrightarrow{HCN} H^+[t\text{-}BuNC.CuBrNC]^- \xrightarrow{C_4H_8} \text{etc.}$$

The infrared data reported[5] for these compounds are the only ones available for copper complexes. By comparison between the infrared CN stretching frequencies of the free t-BuNC and of the complex, the same conclusion can be drawn here as with the silver derivatives.

A not very stable compound containing two molecules of ethyl isocyanide, $CuCN(CNC_2H_5)_2$, was described by Hofmann and Bugge[6], who obtained it by reacting CuCN and C_2H_5NC in ether. Malatesta[7], under analogous experimental conditions, instead obtained a number of compounds containing three molecules of isocyanide: $CuCN(CNR)_3$, where R is ethyl, n-amyl, isoamyl (optically active) or phenyl. A compound of the same type was prepared by Klages and others[8] with p-tolyl isocyanide: $(CuCN(CNC_7H_7)_3$. This compound, when dissolved and then reprecipitated from its solutions, loses a molecule of isocyanide and gives the more stable $CuCN(CNC_7H_7)_2$, thus confirming Hofmann and Bugge's results. It may therefore be concluded that CuCN forms two series of complexes with two and three molecules of isocyanide, respectively, and that the compounds in which copper (I) is coordinately saturated are the least stable and tend to transform into the others by loss of a molecule of ligand. No infrared data are available.

The compounds formed by CuCl with phenyl and p-tolyl isocyanide are very interesting[8]. The relationship among the various products are summarized in Figure 3.2. Compounds 1 are formed by treating a solution of CuCl in aqueous ammonium hydroxide with an excess of isocyanide in alcohol. By careful dilution with water, the products separate in colourless crystals and can be recrystallized from water. They are uni–univalent electrolytes. On boiling in water, compounds **1** give off part of the isocyanide and are transformed into **3**. By dissolving in chloroform and reprecipitating with anhydrous ether, compounds **1** give **2**. These can also be obtained directly from CuCl and an excess of isocyanide in chloroform; from the chloroform solution the products separate by addition of anhydrous ether. Compounds **2** are non-electrolytes. When

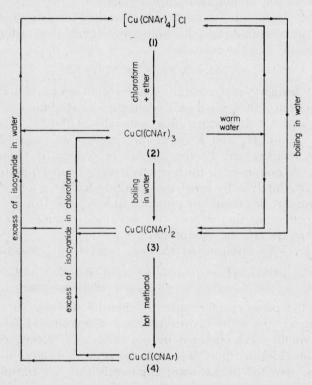

Figure 3.2   Relationships among compounds of CuCl with phenyl and *p*-tolyl isocyanides

treated with water, they rearrange to form compounds **1** and **3**, the former remaining in solution and the latter separating as oils that crystallize on standing. Both compounds **1** and **2** give **3** quantitatively by boiling in water. Compounds **3** can also be prepared directly from CuCl and isocyanides, carrying out the reaction in ether with the required amount of ligand. On recrystallizing from hot methanol, compounds **3** give **4**, which are also slowly formed by CuCl in ether and the calculated amount of isocyanide. Compounds **4** are insoluble in all organic solvents. All these preparations and transformations are shown in Figure 3.2, together with some other obvious relationships among these compounds which are not mentioned in the text.

Copper (II) salts are immediately reduced by aryl isocyanides to copper (I) derivatives, while the isocyanides are transformed into diarylureas and arylammonium chlorides.

Copper was found to catalyse some reactions involving isocyanide. Besides the reaction of addition of hydrogen cyanide to olefin (p. 40), it was found[9] that the reaction:

$$RR'NH + R''NC \rightarrow RR'NCH{=}NR''$$

between primary or secondary amines and isocyanides could be carried out in $\sim 80\%$ yield only when cuprous chloride was present. The reaction temperature was generally $110\text{--}120°$, but when $R = R'' = n\text{-}C_4H_9$ and $R' = H$ the reaction was successful even at room temperature. In the absence of copper (I) chloride the reaction did not proceed; the reagents were recovered quantitatively. Previously, catalysis by fused zinc chloride had been observed and N,N'-di-n-butylformamidine obtained in low yield. It may be noted in this connexion that copper (I) isocyanide complexes are more stable than the zinc (II) complexes.

Similarly, β-γ-unsaturated alcohols react with isocyanide, e.g.,

$$CH_2{=}CHCH_2OH + C_6H_{11}NC \rightarrow CH_2{=}CHCH_2OCH{=}NC_6H_{11}$$
allyl formimidate

only in the presence of copper (I) chloride. Copper (II) chloride gave instead the light brown polymer of cyclohexyl isocyanide; similar results were obtained by use of divalent nickel, cobalt or palladium chloride. Only β-γ-unsaturated alcohol (allyl, methallyl, cinnamyl) reacted in this way; apparently they are complexed by the copper, as evidenced by the lowering of the $\nu(C{=}C)$ in the presence of copper compounds[10].

Silver

Meyer[11] and Gautier[12,13], who first described the preparation of alkyl isocyanides by alkylation of silver cyanide, observed (1856) that compounds of the type AgCN.CNR are formed in the reaction between silver cyanide and alkyl iodides:

$$2\,AgCN + RI \rightarrow AgCN.CNR + AgI$$

As was later shown by Hartley (1916)[14], this reaction proceeds in three stages. At room temperature, the adduct, $AgCN.CH_3I$, is formed, which at 40° reacts to give a product, which, because of its decomposition by water into AgI and CH_3NC, is formulated as iodo(methylisocyano)silver (I). At 100° the last stage of the alkylation reaction of $AgCN$ takes place:

$$AgI(CNCH_3) + AgCN \rightarrow AgI + AgCN(CNCH_3)$$

The same cyano(alkylisocyano)silver compounds are obtained[1] by reacting the corresponding isocyanide with silver cyanide in alcohol, and from potassium alkyl sulphate and potassium dicyanoargentate:

$$K[Ag(CN)_2] + ROSO_3K \rightarrow AgCN(CNR) + K_2SO_4$$

In both cases the products are crystallized from hot alcohol. The $AgCN(CNR)$ compounds are colourless crystalline substances, with a rather high vapour pressure; on standing they first lose their transparency and then turn yellow. On heating they dissociate completely into silver cyanide and isocyanide. The dissociation of $AgCN$-(CNC_2H_5) begins at 60–70° and is complete at about 160°, but above 120° increasing amounts of ethyl cyanide are formed by rearrangement of the isocyanide. Below 120° the mixture contains about 96% of isocyanide, but the total yield is only 16%.

The derivatives of aryl isocyanides are rather unstable. An addition product of phenyl isocyanide and silver cyanide was prepared by W. A. Hofmann (1867)[15] and analysed by K. A. Hofmann (1907)[16]; it was assigned the formula $2 AgCN(CNC_6H_5)$.

More interesting compounds were prepared by Klages and others[18] from p-tolyl isocyanide and a solution of silver nitrate in aqueous ammonium hydroxide at $-20°$. The product, recrystallized from alcohol as colourless needles, has a composition corresponding to $[Ag(CNC_7H_7)_4]NO_3.H_2O$. By addition of ether to a chloroform solution of this compound, the corresponding diisocyanide derivative is formed, viz. $[Ag(CNC_7H_7)_2]NO_3$. The formulation of the complex as a bicoordinate silver (I) complex is in agreement with the infrared spectrum: the bands due to nitrate ion (ca. 1310 and 1390 cm^{-1}, both very broad and strong) are similar to those of the ionic nitrato group. Since the compound is bicoordinate, there is little if any driving force for back donation and, as a consequence, a rise in the CN stretching frequency (ca. 60 cm^{-1}) from the value found in the free isonitrile[17].

The perchlorate of tetrakis(*p*-tolylisocyano)silver $[Ag(CNC_7H_7)_4]$-ClO_4 is analogous to the corresponding nitrate and is obtained at room temperature from an alcoholic solution[18]. In this compound the CN stretching frequency is lower (2177 cm^{-1}) than in $[Ag(CNC_7$-$H_7)_2]NO_3$. Simple dative bonding by four ligands puts much more negative charge on the ligand than that put by two ligands: therefore, there is more electrostatic driving force for back donation with a consequent lowering of the CN frequency[17].

Gold

A number of aryl isocyanide derivatives of gold (I) and gold (III) were prepared by Sacco and Freni[19]. The derivatives of gold (III) were obtained by reacting a cold alcoholic solution of chloroauric (III) acid with aryl isocyanides (two moles per mole of $HAuCl_4$). They are yellow crystalline substances, sparingly soluble in organic solvents, of composition corresponding to $AuCl_3(CNR)$. Their molecular weights were not determined, but in consideration of the dimeric structure of $AuCl_3$[20] they are likely to be monomeric. The trichloro(aryl isocyanide)gold (III) compounds are rather unstable and are spontaneously reduced to the derivatives of gold (I) in the presence of an excess of the isocyanide itself. When the reduction was carried out by warming either the trivalent derivatives or the solution of chloroauric acid with a very large excess of the isocyanide in alcoholic solution, the univalent compounds of formula $[Au(CNR)_4]$-Cl were obtained. These are crystalline substances, stable in the solid state, but unstable in solution unless a large excess of isocyanide is present. The corresponding tetraphenylborate, obtained by exchange reaction with $Na[B(C_6H_5)_4]$ is, however, stable in solution and shows the character of a strong uni–univalent electrolyte.

The cation $[Au(CNR)_4]^+$ is colourless, like the analogous copper and silver ions, and is one of the few examples of coordinately saturated gold (I).

The chlorides of tetrakis(aryl isocyanide)gold (I) can be recrystallized from hot alcohol only in the presence of free isocyanide; otherwise they are transformed into the chlorobis(aryl isocyano)-gold (I) compounds. These were also obtained directly from the gold (III) derivatives, by boiling them in alcohol in the presence of a moderate excess of isocyanide (equal weights of trivalent complex and isocyanide).

The chlorobis(aryl isocyano)gold (I) compounds are yellow,

crystalline substances; soluble in most organic solvents, stable both in the solid state and in solution. Their molecular weights were not determined and their infrared spectra are not available but they are likely to be dimeric with a chlorobridged structure:

$$\begin{array}{ccccc} RNC & & Cl & & CNR \\ \searrow & \swarrow & \diagdown & \swarrow \\ & Au & & Au \\ \nearrow & \diagdown & \nearrow & \nwarrow \\ RNC & & Cl & & CNR \end{array}$$

Other gold (I) complexes are described by Coates[21]. He reacted the polymeric phenylethynylgold (I) with the ligands, in the absence of air, and isolated stable, colourless 1:1 complexes with aliphatic and aromatic isonitriles. The relative donor character of phenyl isocyanide and of other ligands toward phenylethynylgold (I) was established by a series of displacement reactions and was found to be:

$$PEt_3 > P(OPh)_3 > PhNC > AsEt_3 > SbEt_3 > NH_3 > \text{amines} > \text{tertiary}$$
$$\text{amines} > Et_2S = O$$

The CN frequencies of the isocyanide complexes are 80–100 cm^{-1} higher than in the free ligands. The effect, due to the presence of a negative charge on the metal, is expected[17].

Zinc

Isocyanides have a very low affinity for zinc. Their tendency to coordinate to the zinc ion, Zn^{2+}, is lower than for the corresponding amines, and this fact suggested a new method[22] for the separation of the amine–isocyanide mixture which is always obtained in the preparation of isocyanides by the Hofmann method. By reacting ethyl iodide and zinc cyanide, Guillemard obtained[1] a small amount of isocyanide, but did not isolate any addition product.

Some addition compounds of zinc cyanide with alkyl and aryl isocyanides were prepared by Malatesta (1947)[7] by treating $Zn(CN)_2$ with a slight excess of isocyanide. They are colourless powders of formula $Zn(CN)_2(CNR)_2$, where R is n-amyl, isoamyl (optically active), benzyl or phenyl. The derivatives of alkyl isocyanides are water soluble and could not be obtained as crystals; the aromatic derivative is insoluble in water and was obtained in the crystalline state.

The zinc halogenide derivatives of p-tolyl isocyanide, ZnX_2-$(CNC_7H_7)_2$ (X = Cl, Br, I), were prepared[22] by reacting a solution of isocyanide in ether with an ethereal solution of $ZnCl_2$, an aqueous alcohol solution of $ZnBr_2$ and an alcohol solution of ZnI_2, respectively.

Cadmium

The reaction of cadmium cyanide and ethyl iodide was studied by Guillemard who observed the formation of ethyl isocyanide but did not describe any addition product of it with the cadmium salt[1]. Later, Hoelzl studied the methylation of silver tetracyanocadmiate with methyl iodide and of sodium tetracyanocadmiate with dimethyl sulphate[23].

Dry and finely powdered $Ag_2[Cd(CN)_4]$ was shaken for ten days with an excess of CH_3I in the dark at room temperature. The solid mass was extracted with hot methanol; on cooling the solution, a substance separated which, after drying in vacuum, had a composition corresponding to:

$$Cd_4(CN)_4(OH)_4(CNCH_3) . 4 H_2O$$
$$(5)$$

As the presence of the hydroxy groups had to be ascribed to partial hydrolysis, the reaction was repeated excluding any trace of water as carefully as possible. The solid mass obtained under these conditions, recrystallized from water, and dried in vacuum, gave white crystals of composition corresponding to:

$$Cd_2(CN)_2(OH)_2(CNCH_3)$$
$$(6)$$

By shaking a mixture of finely powdered $K_2[Cd(CN)_4]$ with a large excess of dimethyl sulphate for ten days, a liquid and a solid mass were obtained. The solid, extracted with hot anhydrous methanol, gave colourless, water-soluble crystals which analysed as

$$Cd_3(CN)_5(OH)(CNCH_3)_2$$
$$(7)$$

The aqueous solution of this compound reacted alkaline.

The liquid layer, after removal of the excess dimethyl sulphate by distillation under reduced pressure, gave a solid residue which was recrystallized from hot methanol and shown to be a cadmium salt of methyl sulphuric acid, coordinated to isocyanide, possibly

$$Cd(CNCH_3)_4(CH_3SO_4)_2 \quad \text{or} \quad Cd(CNCH_3)_3(CH_3SO_4)_2$$
$$(\textbf{7a}) \qquad\qquad\qquad\qquad (\textbf{7b})$$

The reaction between $K_2[Cd(CN)_4]$ and $(CH_3)_2SO_4$ in molar ratio 1:1 gave instead a product of the formula

$$Cd_6(CN)_{11}(OH)(CNCH_3)$$
$$(8)$$

The results of this research were summarized and interpreted by Hoelzl[23] as follows: the first product formed in the reaction between methyl iodide and silver tetracyanocadmiate is a hypothetical dicyanobis(methylisocyano)cadmium

$$Cd(CN)_2(CNCH_3)_2$$
$$(9)$$

This is unstable and immediately gives off a molecule of isocyanide, thus forming a tricoordinate intermediate (10) which condenses to polynuclear structures with further elimination of isocyanide.

$$(CH_3NC)_2Cd(CN)_2 \rightarrow (CH_3NC)Cd(CN)_2 + CH_3NC$$
$$(9) \qquad\qquad\qquad (10)$$

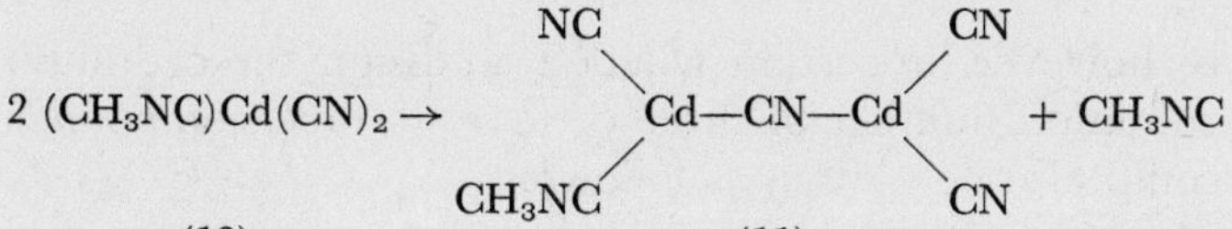

$$2\,(CH_3NC)Cd(CN)_2 \rightarrow \begin{array}{c} NC \\ \diagdown \\ Cd-CN-Cd \\ \diagup \quad\quad \diagdown \\ CH_3NC \quad\quad\quad CN \end{array}{}^{CN}\!\!\diagup \;\; + CH_3NC$$
$$(10) \qquad\qquad\qquad (11)$$

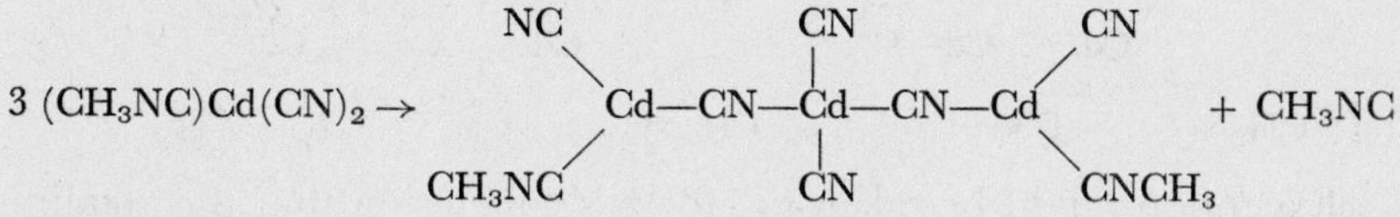

$$3\,(CH_3NC)Cd(CN)_2 \rightarrow \begin{array}{c} NC \\ \diagdown \end{array} \cdots + CH_3NC$$
$$(10) \qquad\qquad\qquad (11a)$$

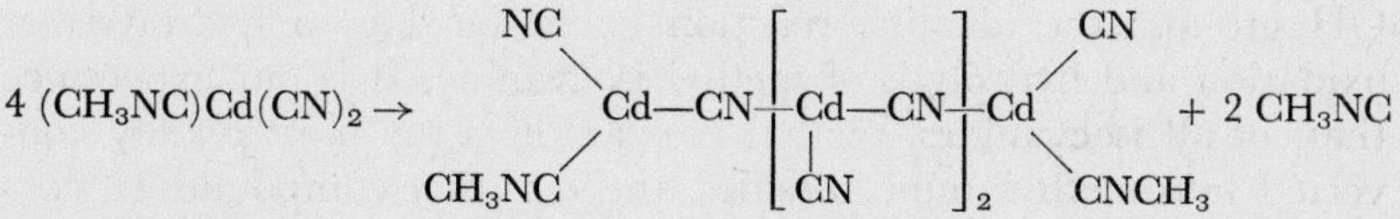

$$4\,(CH_3NC)Cd(CN)_2 \rightarrow \cdots + 2\,CH_3NC$$
$$(10) \qquad\qquad\qquad (12)$$

Compounds 11, 11a and 12 are then hydrolyzed by water to compounds which correspond to 6, 7 and 5, respectively:

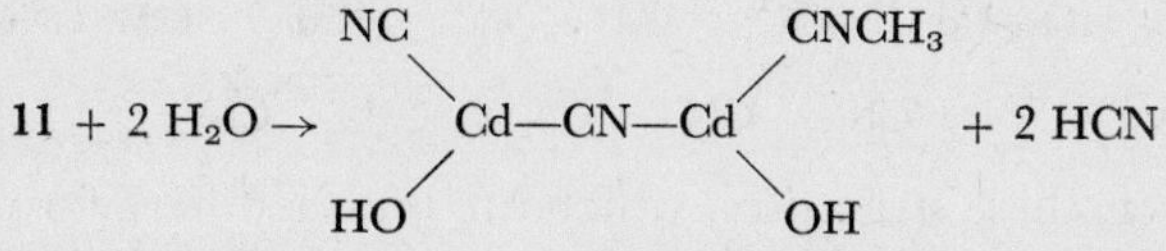

$$11 + 2\,H_2O \rightarrow \begin{array}{c} NC \\ \diagdown \\ Cd-CN-Cd \\ \diagup \quad\quad \diagdown \\ HO \quad\quad\quad OH \end{array}{}^{CNCH_3}\!\!\diagup \;\; + 2\,HCN$$
$$(6)$$

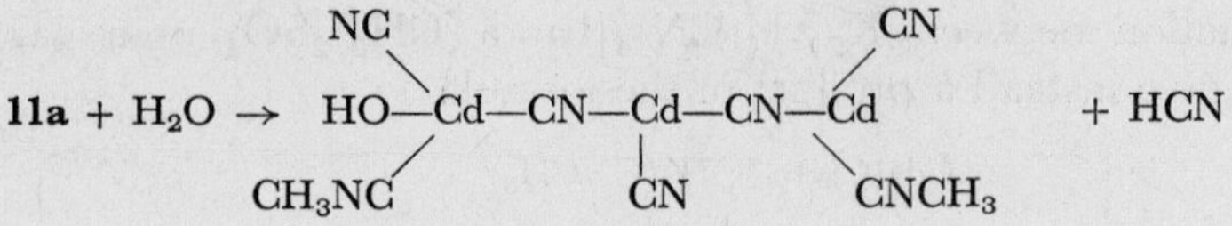

$$\mathbf{11a} + H_2O \rightarrow \overset{\displaystyle NC}{\underset{\displaystyle CH_3NC}{\diagdown\diagup}} HO{-}Cd{-}CN{-}\underset{\displaystyle \underset{\displaystyle CN}{|}}{Cd}{-}CN{-}\overset{\displaystyle CN}{\underset{\displaystyle CNCH_3}{\diagup\diagdown}}Cd \qquad + HCN$$

$$(7)$$

$$\mathbf{12} + 8\,H_2O \rightarrow HO{-}\underset{\displaystyle CH_3NC}{\overset{\displaystyle H_2O}{\diagdown\diagup}}Cd{-}CN{-}\underset{\displaystyle \underset{\displaystyle OH}{|}}{\overset{\displaystyle \overset{\displaystyle H_2O}{|}}{Cd}}{-}CN{-}\underset{\displaystyle \underset{\displaystyle OH}{|}}{\overset{\displaystyle \overset{\displaystyle H_2O}{|}}{Cd}}{-}CN{-}\underset{\displaystyle \underset{\displaystyle OH}{|}}{\overset{\displaystyle \overset{\displaystyle H_2O}{|}}{Cd}}{-}CN + CH_3NC$$

$$+ 4\,HCN$$

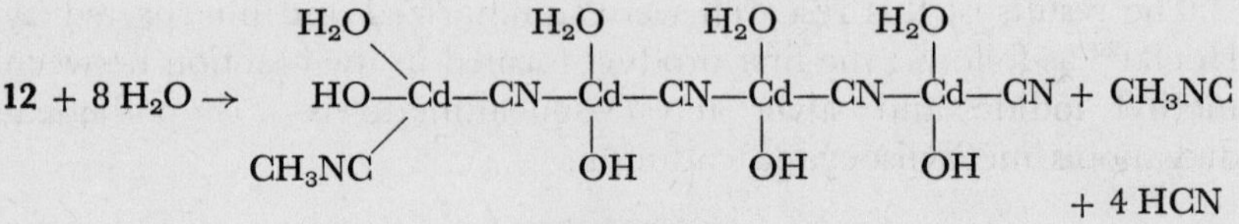

$$(5)$$

Hoelzl thought that the μ-hydroxy forms, which could be postulated as well as the μ-cyano, were to be discarded because (a) the aqueous solutions of **5** and **6** have alkaline reaction, as would be expected for compounds with terminal and not with bridging hydroxy groups; (b) compound **7**, which cannot be formulated as a μ-hydroxy complex, would not fit in with the analogous compounds **5** and **6**.

Hoelzl was, however, uncertain whether to assign the cadmium atoms a coordination number of three or four; in fact, compounds **11** and **11a** could also be written as follows:

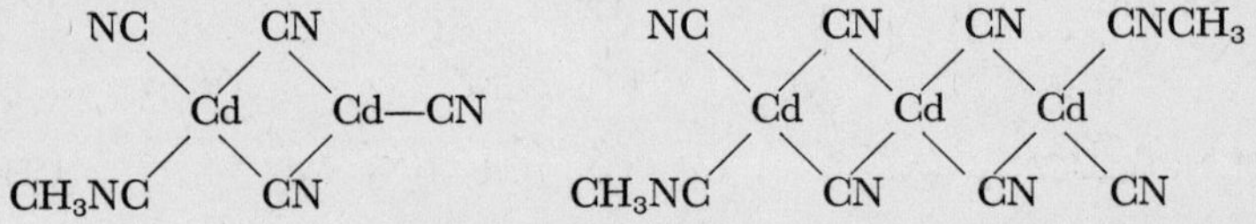

Exception might be taken to Hoelzl's conclusion that the alkaline nature of the compounds is indicative of CN bridges and terminal OH groups; the alkaline reaction could be due to hydrolysis or oxidation and hydrolysis of methyl isocyanide. It is our experience that, of all isocyanides, methyl isocyanide is the most readily converted into methylamine. Besides, the fact that compound **11** does not tend to bind water, not even in diluted aqueous solution, would be better explained by a structure with double cyanide bridges, e.g.

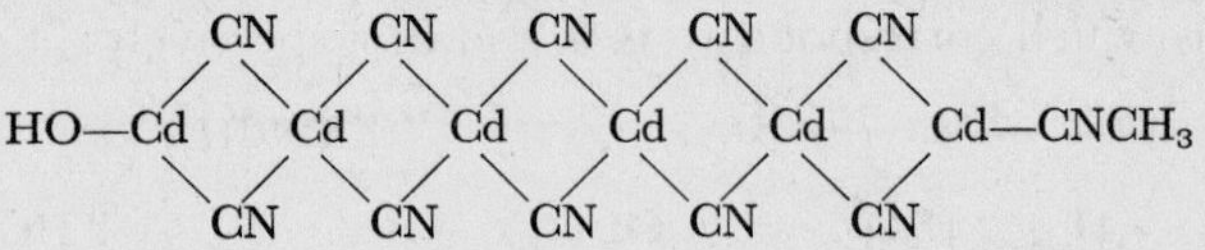

However, these structures, which are reported here for the sake of completeness, were assigned mostly on the basis of analytical evidence.

Clearly, a reinvestigation with the help of modern spectroscopic techniques is needed before any firm conclusion is reached.

Dichloro- and dibromo(p-tolylisocyano)cadmium, $CdCl_2$-(CNC_7H_7) and $CdBr_2(CNC_7H_7)$, were prepared by Sacco[19] and were the only known compounds of cadmium with aryl isocyanides. They are colourless crystalline substances, and were obtained by reacting cadmium halides with an excess of p-tolyl isocyanide in alcohol. Owing to the insolubility of $CdCl_2(CNC_7H_7)$, no molecular weight determination could be carried out. Since similar compounds were not obtained with other cadmium (II) salts, such as the nitrate[24], it is possible that the complex chloride has terminal isocyanide groups ($\nu(CN) \simeq 2200$ cm^{-1}) and bridging chloride groups; a polymer, similar to $CdCl_2$ results and not a monomer or a chloride-bridged dimer, which ought to be soluble in organic solvents.

A remarkable isocyanide complex was obtained by Hieber[25], by reaction of bis(tetracarbonylcobaltate)cadmium (II) with p-anisyl isonitrile in petroleum ether: no carbon monoxide was evolved and a yellow-brown 1 : 2 addition compound was formed. The compound is soluble in organic solvents, except petroleum ether, and is very sensitive to atmospheric oxidation. No other data are available. The possibility that other similar isonitrile complexes are stable means that isonitriles are not very well suited for carbon monoxide displacement for analytical purposes, though this method was used frequently before the advent of i.r. spectroscopy.

Mercury

The reaction between mercuric cyanide, $Hg(CN)_2$, and ethyl iodide was first studied by Guillemard[1] who could not isolate any addition product of the mercuric salt with ethyl isocyanide. Negative results were obtained also by Calmels[26] and by Chwala[27] who affirmed that isocyanides reduce mercuric to mercurous salts, giving no addition products. Later Hartley[28] repeated the reaction between $Hg(CN_2)$ and methyl iodide at 95° and observed a compound of composition corresponding to $HgI_2(CNCH_3)_2$. This product, which could also be obtained from HgI_2 and methyl isocyanide, seemed to contain a dimeric derivative of the isocyanide itself.

Later Klages and others[8] succeeded in preparing the addition product between mercuric chloride and two moles of p-tolyl isocyanide. By treating an ethereal solution of p-tolyl isocyanide cooled to $-20°$, with an ethereal solution of mercuric chloride, the compound $HgCl_2(CNC_7H_7)_2$ separated as colourless crystals, soluble in pyridine and slightly soluble in chloroform. On standing the compound decomposed with separation of Hg_2Cl_2.

When the reaction between isocyanide and $HgCl_2$ is carried out at higher temperature, and with an excess of isocyanide, the latter is oxidized according to the reactions:

$$4 Hg^{2+} + 2 ArNC + 3 H_2O \rightarrow 2 Hg_2^{2+} + (ArNH)_2CO + CO_2 + 4 H^+$$
$$4 H_2O + 4 H^+ + 4 ArNC + 4 ROH \rightarrow 4 ArNH_2^+ + 4 HCO_2R$$

The formation of aryl isocyanide complexes of the cadmium carbonylmetallates, as for example, $(ArNC)_2Cd[Co(CO)_4]_2$, is not paralleled by a similar reactivity of the mercury compounds. As with other mercury isonitrile complexes, the stability is lower here than with cadmium or zinc. Both bis(tetracarbonylcobalt)mercury (II)[25] and bis(tricarbonylnitrosyliron)mercury (II)[29] are decomposed by isocyanides, just as they are by other bases, yielding $[Co(RNC)_5]$ $[Co(CO)_4]$ or $[Fe(RNC)_6]$ $[Fe(NO)(CO)_3]_2$ respectively.

ISOCYANIDE COMPOUNDS OF OTHER TYPICAL ELEMENTS

Only Group III elements are known to yield stable complexes with isocyanide ligands. These complexes give chemical evidence of the ability of isocyanide to act as a simple donor.

While the 1:1 complexes of boron are rather reactive, since the tendency to further reaction gives interesting boron–nitrogen heterocycles or polymers, the only complexes reported so far for aluminium or the lanthanides have no tendency to give similar reactions.

Boron

Strong Lewis acids, such as trialkyl or triarylboron compounds should, in principle, be capable of giving 1:1 adducts with isocyanides, as the latter are weak Lewis bases. The existence of such 1:1 adducts was proved by Casanova[30,31], who obtained white crystalline, volatile t-BuNC.BMe_3, in quantitative yields by mixing the reagents in the presence or in the absence of ethyl ether. The evidence in favour of the proposed structure includes the ${}^1H$ n.m.r. spectrum. In $CHCl_3$ at $-20°$ the C-methyl resonances are at 8·55 ($J_{NH} = 2·0$ cps) and the B-methyl resonances at $\tau = 10·12$ (no B–H coupling constant is reported). The appearance of the triplet due to N–H spin–spin splitting was assumed to indicate a high degree of symmetry around the nitrogen atom, as in the parent free ligand; this splitting was not observed with less symmetrical compounds, such as $[(RCH_2NC)_5Fe(CN)]^+$ salts[32]. The infrared spectrum presents a strong CN band, as required by a bond order higher here than in the free ligand. The mass spectrum was also obtained as is in accord with the proposed structure. The complex is not very stable; on long standing in an evacuated tube it is transformed into another compound, which is air stable and not very volatile, m.p. 119–120°:

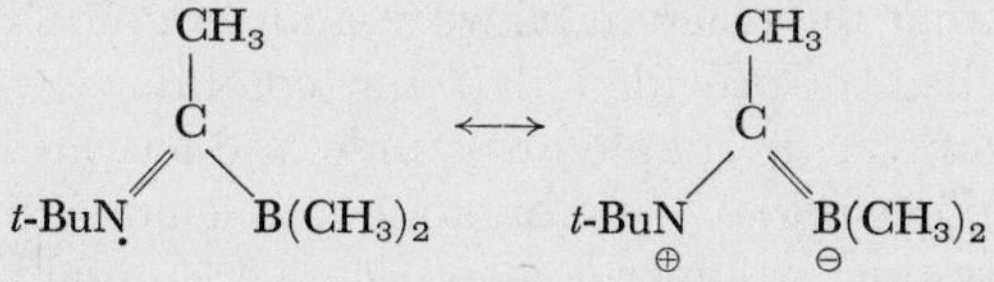

Two other white 1:1 adducts were obtained from triethylboron and ethyl isocyanide in anhydrous ether at 20°[33,34,35]. However, the molecular weights (which indicated a dimer) and the absence of any absorption band in the 1650–2500 cm^{-1} region ruled out a similar formula. The results of the investigation favour the following formulae, **13** and **14**, for the two compounds:

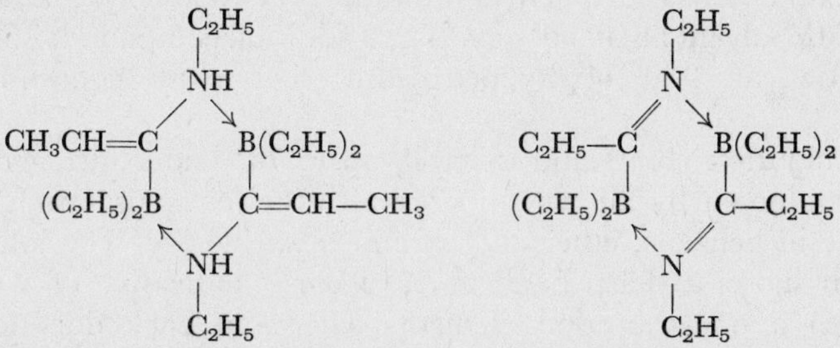

(13)   (14)

Another compound with a structure similar to **14** had been obtained by Hesse, from phenyl isocyanide and triethyl- or tributyl-boron[36]. Later Hesse[37] extended the reaction to many other isocyanides and triorganoboron compounds, always with the same results.

The reaction is likely to go through the intermediate formation of a 1:1 adduct. Besides the already mentioned $(CH_3)_3B.CNC-(CH_3)_3$, similar adducts were isolated with triphenylboron; some of these complexes were rather stable. On heating, 2,5-diboradihydropyrazine derivatives were formed[38,39].

The reaction between diborane and phenylisocyanide was reported to yield

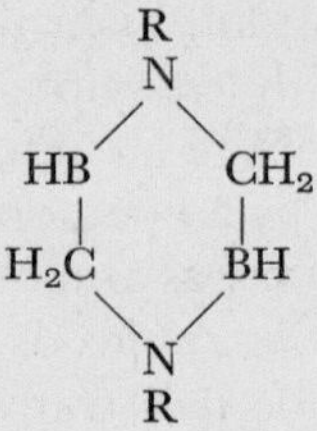

$$
\begin{array}{c}
\overset{\displaystyle R}{\underset{\displaystyle N}{}} \\
HB \diagup \quad \diagdown CH_2 \\
H_2C \quad \quad BH \\
\diagdown N \diagup \\
R
\end{array}
$$

However, Bresadola and others failed to isolate such a compound. They found[34] that the reaction between an isocyanide and diborane offered no difficulty, provided that the conditions were carefully controlled. However no simple isocyanide adduct was formed[35]. By reaction of diisocyanides with organoboron compounds or boron hydrides interesting polymeric materials were obtained. Some of these polymers were soluble in organic solvents when the average molecular weight was 10,000–12,000, while those with higher molecular weight were insoluble.

Aluminium

The reaction between triphenylaluminium and cyclohexyl isocyanide in aromatic solvent at 50–60° gave a 1:1 addition compound, isolated by addition at $-20°$ of dry petroleum ether to the concentrated solution[40].

The colourless compound is stable up to 75° under nitrogen but it is decomposed by air with liberation of cyclohexylisocyanide. It is soluble in benzene, ether and carbon tetrachloride. The infrared spectrum shows a sharp band at 2215 cm^{-1} indicative of a complex with a non-transition element, where no back donation is possible.

The same compound was also obtained[40] by another synthesis:

$$Ph_3BL + AlEt_3 \rightarrow BEt_3 + Ph_3AlL \quad (L = C_6H_{11}NC)$$

No evidence for a reactivity like that found for the boron adducts was reported for this complex.

Lanthanides

Isonitrile derivatives of lathanide elements were described only in 1966 by E. O. and H. Fischer[41]. The crystalline, air- and moisture-sensitive complexes (see Table 3.5) were prepared by the quantitative reaction between cyclohexylisonitrile and tricyclopentadienylmetal in benzene at room temperature. The compounds are thermally stable up to 240°, and are soluble in organic solvents; they can be sublimed with only slight loss due to decomposition. The compounds are quite similar to other addition compounds of the tricyclopentadienyls, such as $(C_5H_5)_3M.THF$ (M = Eu, Tb, Ho, Yb) or $(C_5H_5)_3Yb.NH_3$. The bond between the ligand and the lanthanide metal is a σ-bond, as shown by the position of the infrared band due to the CN stretching (see Table 3.5). The bond between the metal and the cyclopentadienyl ring is considered to be covalent, and not ionic. Strong bands observed in the region 600–660 cm^{-1} may be assigned to ring–metal vibrations. Further, the CH deformation band, at 780–794 cm^{-1} is at higher frequency than in the ionic alkali-metal cyclopentadienides.

Group IVB elements

No isocyanide complex of this group has been reported. The possibility that some trisorganometal cyanide might actually be the iso-compound was discussed in the literature, but no definite evidence for this is available.

Ebsworth[43] ruled out the presence of more than small amounts of isocyanide in equilibrium with the cyanide at room temperature in the case of SiH_3CN and all three $SiH_x(CH_3)_yCN$ ($x + y = 3$).

A paper by Seyferth[44] gives a summary of the various available lines of evidence for $R_3M(CN)$. Trimethyltin (IV) cyanide shows rather polar properties while trimethyl(iso)cyanogermane and trimethyl(iso)cyanosilane and covalent molecules. For the latter compounds evidence was found to show that they are equilibrium mixtures of cyano- and isocyanide-derivative, with the former isomer predominating.

Stable compounds where an isocyanide group is bonded to a Group IV element are known. Trisorganotin (IV) and trisorganosilicon (IV) isocyanide complexes of iron, chromium, molybdenum and tungsten were described by Seyferth[45] and by King[46]. The complexes, which will be described under the appropriate transition metal, afford further examples of stabilization of unstable species by complex formation.

Table 3.1   Isocyanide compounds of copper

Name	Formula[a]	Colour and crystal form	M.p. or dec. temp., °C	I.r. data	Ref.
Bromo(methyl isocyanide)copper(I)	$CuBr(CNCH_3)$	White crystals			3
Iodo(methyl isocyanide)copper(I)	$CuI(CNCH_3)$	White needles			2,3
Iodo(ethyl isocyanide)copper(I)	$CuI(CNC_2H_5)$	Colourless needles			3
Cyano(ethyl isocyanide)copper(I)	$Cu(CN)(CNC_2H_5)$	Big colourless prisms			1
Iodo(n-propyl isocyanide)copper(I)	$CuI(CNC_3H_7)$	Colourless needles			3
Cyano(n-propyl isocyanide)copper(I)	$Cu(CN)(CNC_3H_7)$	Big colourless rhombic tables			1
Cyano(isobutyl isocyanide)copper(I)	$Cu(CN)(CNC_4H_9)$	Big colourless rhombic prisms			1
Chloro(phenyl isocyanide)copper(I)	$CuCl(CNC_6H_5)$	White needles	184–185		8
Cyanobis(ethyl isocyanide)copper(I)	$Cu(CN)(CNC_2H_5)_2$	—	128		6
Chlorobis(phenyl isocyanide)copper(I)	$CuCl(CNC_6H_5)_2$	White needles	128		8
Cyanobis(phenyl isocyanide)copper(I)	$Cu(CN)(CNC_6H_5)_2$	White flakes	158–162		8
Cyanotris(ethyl isocyanide)copper(I)	$Cu(CN)(CNC_2H_5)_3$	Brown crystals			7
Bromotris(t-butyl isocyanide)copper(I)	$CuBr(CNC_4H_9)_3$	Colourless needles	151–153	2182	5
Cyanotris(t-butyl isocyanide)copper(I)	$CuCN(CNC_4H_9)_3$	Colourless needles	196–198	{2182, 2140}	5
Cyanotris(n-amyl isocyanide)copper(I)	$Cu(CN)(CNC_5H_{11})_3$	—			7
Cyanotris(isoamyl isocyanide)copper(I)	$Cu(CN)(CNC_5H_{11})_3$	—			7
Chlorotris(phenyl isocyanide)copper(I)	$CuCl(CNC_6H_5)_3$	Colourless crystals	156		8
Cyanotris(phenyl isocyanide)copper(I)	$Cu(CN)(CNC_6H_5)_3$	White crystals	126–128		7, 8
Chlorotris(p-tolyl isocyanide)copper(I)	$CuCl(CNC_7H_7)_3$	Colourless crystals	170–172		8
Chlorotris(p-tolyl isocyanide)copper(I) with one mole ethanol	$[CuCl(CNC_7H_7)_3 \cdot C_2H_5OH]$	Colourless prisms	170		8
Phenylacetylenide-tris(p-tolyl isocyanide)copper(I)	$Cu(CNC_7H_7)_3C_2C_6H_5$	White needles	100 (dec.)		8
Tetrakis(phenyl isocyanide)copper(I) chloride hexahydrate	$[Cu(CNC_6H_5)_4]Cl.6\,H_2O$	Colourless needles	102		8
Tetrakis(p-tolyl isocyanide)copper(I) chloride monohydrate	$[Cu(CNC_7H_7)_4]Cl.H_2O$	Colourless crystals	127		8
Tetrakis(p-tolyl isocyanide)copper(I) perchlorate	$[Cu(CNC_7H_7)_4]ClO_4$	White needles	175		22

[a] Whenever the structure of the compound was not reported by the author and cannot be unambiguously deduced, the simplest name and formula were adopted.

Table 3.2 Isocyanide compounds of silver and gold

Name	Formula[a]	Colour and crystals form	M.p. or dec. temp. °C	Other data	Ref.
Isocyanide compounds of silver					
Cyano(methyl isocyanide)silver (t)	AgCN(CNCH₃)	Colourless needles	75–76	+7·0[f]	1
Cyano(ethyl isocyanide)silver (t)	AgCN(CNC₂H₅)	Colourless needles	96–97	+6·9[f]	1
Cyano(n-propyl isocyanide)silver (t)	AgCN(CNC₃H₇)	Colourless needles	—	+6·7[f]	1
Cyano(isobutyl isocyanide)silver (t)	AgCN(CNC₄H₉)	Colourless needles	—	+5·9[f]	1
Cyano(isoamyl isocyanide)silver (t)	AgCN(CNC₅H₁₁)	Colourless needles	—	+4·45[f]	1
Bis(p-tolyl isocyanide)silver (t) nitrate	[Ag(CNC₇H₇)₂]NO₃	White crystals	122–123	[d]	8
Tetrakis(p-tolyl isocyanide)silver (t) nitrate monohydrate	[Ag(CNC₇H₇)₄]NO₃·H₂O	White crystals	100–103		8
Tetrakis(p-tolyl isocyanide)silver (t) perchlorate	[Ag(CNC₇H₇)₄]ClO₄	White crystals	101	[e]	22
Isocyanide compounds of gold					
Chlorophenyl isocyanide gold (t)	AuCl(CNC₆H₅)	White crystals	—		19
Chloro(p-tolyl isocyanide)gold (t)	AuCl(CNC₇H₇)	White crystals	—		19
Cyano(p-tolyl isocyanide)gold (t)	Au(CN)(CNC₇H₇)	White crystals	244 (dec.)		19
Chloro(p-anisyl isocyanide)gold (t)	AuCl(CNC₇H₇O)	White crystals	—		19
Tetrakis(phenyl isocyanide)gold (t) chloride	[Au(CNC₆H₅)₄]Cl	White crystals	190		19
Tetrakis(p-tolyl isocyanide)gold (t) chloride	[Au(CNC₇H₇)₄]Cl	White crystals	175 (dec.)		19
Tetrakis(p-tolyl isocyanide)gold (t) tetraphenylborate	[Au(CNC₇H₇)₄]Ph₄B	White needles	—		19
Tetrakis(p-anisyl isocyanide)gold (t) chloride	[Au(CNC₇H₇O)₄]Cl	Colourless needles	40·5–41·5	[a]	21
(n-butyl isocyanide)phenylethynylgold (t)	Au(C₈H₅)(CNC₄H₉)	Colourless leaflets	176–177 (dec.)	[b]	21
(p-tolyl isocyanide)phenylethynylgold (t)	Au(C₈H₅)(CNC₇H₇)	Colourless needles	107–108 (dec.)	—	21
(o-ethylphenyl isocyanide)phenylethynylgold (t)	Au(C₈H₅)(CNC₈H₉)	Colourless needles	107–108	[c]	21
Trichloro(p-tolyl isocyanide)gold (m)	AuCl₃(CNC₇H₇)	Yellow crystals	—		19
Trichloro(p-anisyl isocyanide)gold (m)	AuCl₃(CNC₇H₇O)	Yellow crystals	—		19

[a] I.r. spectrum (KBr): 2130, 2249 (CN). In CCl₄:2134 and 2253 cm⁻¹
[b] I.r. spectrum (KBr): no C≡C stretching visible, 2232 (CN),
[c] I.r. spectrum: no C≡C stretching, 2218 (KBr) or 2211 (C₆H₆).
[d] CN stretching frequency (CHCl₃): 2195·7.
[e] CN stretching frequencies (CHCl₃):2186 sh, 2177s, 2136w.[17]
[f] Molar heats of formation of AgCN + RNC, in Kcal/mole[1].

Table 3.3 Isocyanide compounds of the elements of group IIB

Name	Formula	Colour and crystal form	M.p.	Note	Ref.
		Isocyanide complexes of zinc			
Dicyanobis(n-amyl isocyanide)zinc (II)	$Zn(CN)_2(CNC_5H_{11})_2$	Golden yellow powder	—	—	7
Dicyanobis(isoamyl isocyanide)zinc (II)	$Zn(CN)_2(CNC_5H_{11})_2$	Golden yellow powder	—	—	7
Dicyanobis(phenyl isocyanide)zinc (II)	$Zn(CN)_2(CNC_6H_5)_2$	Golden yellow crystals	—	—	7
Dicyanobis(benzyl isocyanide)zinc (II)	$Zn(CN)_2(CNC_7H_7)_2$	Golden yellow powder	—	—	7
Dichlorobis(p-tolyl isocyanide)zinc (II)	$ZnCl_2(CNC_7H_7)_2$	White crystals	146	—	22
Dibromobis(p-tolylisocyanide)zinc (II)	$ZnBr_2(CNC_7H_7)_2$	White needles	166 (dec.)	—	22
Diiodobis(p-tolyl isocyanide)zinc (II)	$ZnI_2(CNC_7H_7)_2$	Pale yellow needles	155–160	—	22
		Isocyanide compounds of cadmium[a]			
Dichloro(p-tolyl isocyanide)cadmium (II)	$CdCl_2(CNC_7H_7)$	White crystals	270 (dec.)	b	19, 24
Dibromo(p-tolyl isocyanide)cadmium (II)	$CdBr_2(CNC_7H_7)$	Dirty white	170 (dec.)	—	19
Bis(tetracarbonylcobaltato)bis(p-anisylisonitrile)cadmium (II)	$Cd[Co(CO)_4]_2(CNC_7H_7O)_2$	Yellow-brown	—	c	25
		Isocyanide compounds of mercury			
Dichloro(p-tolyl isocyanide)mercury (II)	$HgCl_2(CNC_7H_7)_2$	Colourless crystals	unstable at room temp.	—	8

[a] Hoelzl's compounds are not tabulated.
[b] CN stretching frequency: 2184 cm^{-1} in nujol[24].
[c] Very air sensitive.

Table 3.4   Isocyanide compounds of boron

Name	Formula	Dec. point	ν(CN)	Ref.
Triphenylboron cyclohexyl isocyanide	$(C_6H_5)_3B.CNC_6H_{11}$	126–128	2255	39
Triphenylboron isopropyl isocyanide	$(C_6H_5)_3B.CNC_3H_7$	105–108	2265	39
Triphenylboron t-butyl isocyanide	$(C_6H_5)_3B.CNC_4H_9$	150–155	2275	39
Triphenylboron n-butyl isocyanide	$(C_6H_5)_3B.CNC_4H_9$	94–97	2255	39
Triphenylboron phenyl isocyanide	$(C_6H_5)_3B.CNC_6H_5$	75–85	2225	39
Triphenylboron 4-diethylaminophenyl isocyanide	$(C_6H_5)_3B(CNC_{10}H_{16}N)$	109–111	2245	39
Trimethylboron methyl isocyanide[a]	$(CH_3)_3B.CNCH_3$	68–70	2247	30

[a] Partial H n.m.r. data and mass spectrum are available[30].

Table 3.5   Isocyanide compounds of lanthanides

Compounds	Colour	M.p.	ν(CN)[a]	Magnetic moment (B.M.) found[b]	theory
$(C_5H_5)_3Y(CNC_6H_{11})$	colourless	165	2208	0	0
$(C_5H_5)_3Nd(CNC_6H_{11})$	violet	147	2207	3·4	3·7
$(C_5H_5)_3Tb(CNC_6H_{11})$	colourless	162	2205	10·1	9·7
$(C_5H_5)_3Ho(CNC_6H_{11})$	yellow	165	2203	10·6	10·4
$(C_5H_5)_3Yo(CNC_6H_{11})$	dark green	167	—	4·4	4·5

[a] Nujol-hostaflon, all strong bands.
[b] Determined in benzene solution, according to Evans' method[42].

REFERENCES

1. H. Guillemard, *Ann. Chim. Phys.*, [VIII] **14**, 344 (1908).
2. E. J. G. Hartley, *J. Chem. Soc.*, **1928**, 780.
3. H. Irving and M. Jonason, *J. Chem. Soc.*, **1960**, 2095.
4. P. J. Fischer, N. E. Taylor and M. M. Harding, *J. Chem. Soc.*, **1960**, 2303.
5. S. Otsuka, K. Mori and K. Yamagami, *J. Org. Chem.*, **31**, 4170 (1966).
6. K. A. Hofmann and G. Bugge, *Chem. Ber.*, **40**, 1772 (1907).
7. L. Malatesta, *Gazz. Chim. Ital.*, **77**, 340 (1957).
8. F. Klages, K. Moenkemeyer and R. Heinle, *Chem. Ber.*, **85**, 109 (1952).
9. T. Saegusa, Y. Ito, S. Kobayashi, K. Irota and H. Yoshiota, *Tetrahedron Letters*, **1966**, 6121.
10. T. Saegusa, Y. Ito, S. Kobayashi and K. Hirota, *Tetrahedron Letters*, **1967**, 521
11. E. Meyer, *J. Prakt. Chem.*, [1] **68**, 279 (1856).
12. M. Gautier, *Ann. Chim. Phys.*, [IV] **17**, 203 (1869).
13. M. Gautier, *Ann. Chim. Phys.*, [IV] **17**, 222 (1869).
14. E. G. J. Hartley, *J. Chem. Soc.*, **109**, 1296 (1916).
15. W. A. Hofmann, *Ann. Chim. Phys.*, [IV] **17**, 210 (1869).
16. K. A. Hofmann and G. Bugge, *Chem. Ber.*, **40**, 1772 (1907).
17. F. A. Cotton and F. Zingales, *J. Am. Chem. Soc.*, **83**, 351 (1961).
18. A. Sacco, *Gazz. Chim. Ital.*, **84**, 370 (1954).
19. A. Sacco and M. Freni, *Gazz. Chim. Ital.*, **86**, 195 (1956).
20. W. Fischer, *Z. anorg. Chem.*, **176**, 81 (1928).
21. G. E. Coates and C. Parkin, *J. Chem. Soc.*, **1962**, 3220.

22. A. Sacco, *Gazz. Chim. Ital.*, **85**, 989 (1955).
23. F. Hoelzl, *Monatsh.*, **51**, 402 (1929).
24. Unpublished results.
25. W. Hieber and R. Breu, *Chem. Ber.*, **90**, 1259 (1957).
26. G. Calmels, *Compt. Rend.*, **99**, 239 (1884).
27. A. Chwala, *Angew. Chem.*, **20**, 1366 (1907).
28. E. G. J. Hartley, *J. Chem. Soc.*, **109**, 1302 (1916).
29. W. Hieber and W. Klingshirn, *Z. anorg. Chem.*, **323**, 292 (1963).
30. J. Casanova and R. E. Schuster, *Tetrahedron Letters*, **1964**, 405.
31. J. Casanova, H. R. Kiefer, D. Kuwada and A. H. Boulton, *Tetrahedron Letters*, **1965**, 703.
32. W. Z. Heldt, *Inorg. Chem.*, **2**, 1048 (1963).
33. S. Bresadola, G. Carraro, C. Pecile and A. Turco, *Tetrahedron Letters*, **1964**, 3185.
34. S. Bresadola, G. Rossetto and G. Puosi, *Gazz. Chim. Ital.*, **96**, 1397 (1966).
35. S. Bresadola, G. Rossetto and G. Puosi, *Tetrahedron Letters*, **1965**, 4775.
36. G. Hesse and H. Witte, *Angew. Chem.*, **75**, 791 (1963); *Angew. Chem. (Int. Edit.)*, **2**, 617 (1963).
37. G. Hesse and H. Witte, *Annalen*, **687**, 1 (1965).
38. G. Hesse, H. Witte and W. Gulden, *Tetrahedron Letters*, **1966**, 2707.
39. G. Hesse, W. Witte and G. Bittner, *Annalen*, **687**, 9 (1965).
40. G. Hesse, H. Witte and P. Mischke, *Angew. Chem.*, **77**, 380 (1965); *Angew. Chem. (Int. Edit.)*, **4**, 355 (1965).
41. E. O. Fischer and H. Fischer, *J. Organomet. Chem.*, **6**, 141 (1966).
42. D. F. Evans, *J. Chem. Soc.*, **1959**, 2002.
43. E. A. V. Ebsworth and S. G. Frankiss, *J. Chem. Soc.*, **1963**, 661.
44. D. Seyferth and N. Kahlen, *J. Org. Chem.*, **25**, 809 (1960).
45. D. Seyferth and N. Kahlen, *J. Am. Chem. Soc.*, **82**, 1080 (1960).
46. R. B. King, *Inorg. Chem.*, **6**, 25 (1967).

4 ISOCYANIDE COMPLEXES OF GROUP VI ELEMENTS

Zerovalent isocyanide complexes are known for all the elements of the group, but those of chromium and molybdenum are better known than those of tungsten, as the latter are rather difficult to obtain. Ionic complexes with isocyanide ligands in the anionic part are stable only in the case of tungsten. Trivalent chromium complexes of isocyanides as well as the related Mo^{IV} and W^{IV} compounds have been described, but all of them are ill-defined. No infrared or other physical data are available for these compounds.

CHROMIUM

Derivatives of Chromium (III)

The affinity of chromium (III) for isocyanides is extremely poor, and the addition compounds between chromium (III) salts and isocyanides, if ever they form, are immediately decomposed by water.

Hoelzl[1] studied the alkylation of $K_3[Cr(CN)_6]$ with dimethyl sulphate and of $Ag_3[Cr(CN)_6]$ with methyl iodide. In this way he could only obtain mixtures of what appeared to be polynuclear products, probably with bridging CN groups, containing some molecules of isocyanides. In Hoelzl's opinion, the first product formed during the course of the reaction is a hypothetical 'methyl-chromiumcyanide', that is, a tricyanotris(methylisocyano)chromium (III), which immediately loses hydrocyanic acid and methyl isocyanide to give a still hypothetical dinuclear compound:

$$
\begin{array}{ccc}
CH_3NC & CN & CN \\
\searrow & \searrow\nearrow & \nearrow \\
CH_3NC\rightarrow Cr & -CN\rightarrow Cr & -CN \\
\nearrow & \nearrow\searrow & \searrow \\
CH_3NC & CN & CN
\end{array}
$$

By hydrolysis this gives the products actually observed in the reaction, which were written as:

$$
\begin{array}{ccc}
CH_3NC & CN & CN \\
\searrow & \searrow\nearrow & \nearrow \\
H_2O\rightarrow Cr & -CN\rightarrow Cr & -OH \\
\nearrow & \nearrow\searrow & \\
H_2O & CN & OH
\end{array}
\qquad
\begin{array}{ccc}
CH_3NC & CN & OH \\
\searrow & \searrow\nearrow & \nearrow \\
H_2O\rightarrow Cr & -CN\rightarrow Cr & -OH \\
\nearrow & \nearrow\searrow & \\
H_2O & CN & OH
\end{array}
$$

The latter was also isolated as a dihydrate and a pentahydrate. These products are soluble in water and very difficult to crystallize; their identification is not completely satisfactory, and the formulae proposed by Hoelzl do not seem sufficiently proved.

Derivatives of Cr (0)

Compounds with isocyanides as the only ligands

Hexa(arylisocyanide)chromium compounds, $Cr(CNAr)_6$, formally derived from chromium carbonyl, were obtained by Malatesta and coworkers[2,3]. When an alcoholic suspension of chromium (II) acetate is treated with an excess of arylisocyanide, a lively reaction occurs, which has to be considered as a disproportionation of Cr^{II} to Cr^{III} and Cr^0 and may be written as follows:

$$3\,Cr^{2+} + 18\,RNC \rightarrow Cr(CNR)_6 + 2\,[Cr(CNR)_6]^{3+}$$

The hexa(arylisocyanide)chromium (III) salts could not be isolated, but the yield of $Cr(CNR)_6$ agrees with the above equation.

By reacting 3 moles of $Cr(CH_3COO)_2$ with 6 moles of C_6H_5NC, 0·309 mole of $Cr(CNC_6H_5)_6$ was obtained and 1·77 moles of $Cr(CH_3COO)_2$ remained in the solution. The same reaction, repeated with 3 moles of chromium (II) acetate and 18 moles of isocyanide, gave 0·945 mole of $Cr(CNC_6H_5)_6$.

An alternative route to hexa(arylisocyanide)chromium (o) from tris(dipyridyl)chromium(o) and excess isonitrile afforded only an 11% yield[4]. The low yield is not due to an unfavourable equilibrium: the isonitrile complex is unaffected by dipyridyl below the temperature of decomposition.

Hexa(arylisocyanide)chromium compounds are diamagnetic, crystalline substances, of colours varying from yellow to red with green or metallic reflectances. They are quite stable to air and melt without decomposition in a rather high temperature range (125–200°). They are soluble in chloroform and benzene, sparingly soluble in alcohol and insoluble in water. The solutions are stable to air in the cold, but decompose on prolonged boiling. Hexa(arylisocyanide)-chromium compounds are slowly decomposed by aqueous solutions of strong mineral acids, but are not affected by alkali, not even by hot sodium alcoholate. However they react with trialkylaluminium and the reaction product is an effective catalyst for obtaining iso-tactic 1,2-polybutadiene[5,6].

Kinetic measurements are in agreement with the observed stability of the complexes. The rate of the exchange of $Cr(CNC_6H_5)_6$ with ^{14}C-labelled phenyl isonitrile has been studied at 20° and 75° in benzene solution[7]. The exchange reaction at 20° is rather slow, the half-life being some hundreds of hours. The first-order rate constants are 0·028 at 20° and 0·210 sec^{-1} at 75°. The reaction is first order in the complex and zero order in the ligand, in agreement with an S_N1 dissociative mechanism, as found for the exchange between carbon monoxide and chromium hexacarbonyl. The rate is lower for the isonitrile than for the carbonyl complexes in agreement with the lowering of the energy of the metal–carbon bond due to the lower contribution from back-donation in the isonitrile complexes[7].

The infrared spectra of the compounds were studied by Cotton and Zingales[8] in $CHCl_3$ solution. The presence of more than one CN stretching frequency was taken as evidence for distortion of the molecule from octahedral symmetry (which would require only one i.r. active band). The reason for the distortion was then thought to be a significant contribution by **1** (p. 25) to the resonance hybrid, with the consequent bending of each C–N–C grouping.

A significant contribution by **1** also requires a depression of the CN stretching frequency going from the free ligand to the complex: indeed a depression of 60–200 cm^{-1} was observed. More recent work by Cotton[9] showed, however, that in terminal CNR groups there is no evidence for a CNC angle significantly different from 180° in all the reliable x-ray structure determinations carried out up to now. Therefore the recorded infrared spectra have to be explained as due to the distortion of bulky arylisocyanide groups. The lowering of the CN stretching frequency can be explained, as with chromium hexacarbonyl, by back-donation.

Compounds with carbonyl ligands

An accurate description of the conditions in which the various $M(CO)_{6-n}(RCN)_n$ compounds are formed (n = 1, 2, 3; M = Cr, Mo, W) was given by Murdoch[10]. By reaction of tetraethylammonium iodopentacarbonylmetal in tetrahydrofuran with isonitrile in a 75 foot vacuum, the starting complex disappeared after 3–5 hours at room temperature or at 45° (M = W). The monoisonitrile complex was removed by sublimation and the residue contained nearly pure bis(isocyanide)complex. Substitution of the chloro- for the iododerivative as starting material afforded a mixture of all the three possible substitution products (M = Cr, Mo), which were then separated fractionally, the monosubstituted one being present only in small quantity.

The variables influencing the reaction (probably of S_N2 type) were also studied. An increase of carbon monoxide pressure or of the concentration of halide ion decreased the reaction rate. The nature of the isocyanide was not decisive on the reaction rate, although the formation of the trisubstituted product was favoured with phenylisocyanide. The influence of the anion (Cl$^-$ vs. I$^-$) was as remarkable as found with $Mn(CO)_5X$. A mechanism was proposed for the reaction (Figure 4.1). Additional support was found in the actual isolation of two ionic intermediates in the case of tungsten complexes,

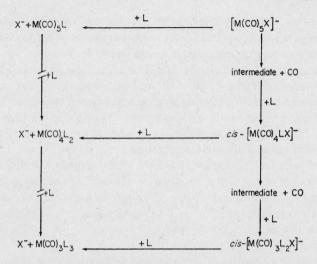

Figure 4.1   Mechanism for a reaction leading to Group VI
carbonyl isocyanide complexes

and in the lack of reactivity of mono- and disubstituted compounds
towards excess ligand.

Direct substitution of carbonyl groups in $Cr(CO)_6$ was found
possible, but only a monosubstituted product was obtained and a
temperature of 120–130° was required[11]. Similarly, pentacarbonyl-
(phenylisocyanide)chromium was obtained in toluene solution,
together with unreacted starting material[12].

Disubstituted products are best prepared by refluxing a benzene
solution of tetracarbonyl(1,5-cyclooctadiene)chromium with the
appropriate ligand: the reported infrared spectrum[12] suggests a *cis*
configuration for the compound with phenylisocyanide. On the
other hand the complex reported by Strohmeier[13], $(CO)_4(NCC_6-H_{11})_2Cr$, must have a *trans* configuration, since it has no appreciable
dipole moment.

Disubstituted compounds are kinetically stable; an attempt to
convert the *cis*-isomer to *trans*- by heating its solution resulted only
in disproportionation

$$2\,Mo(CO)_4L_2 \rightarrow Mo(CO)_5L + Mo(CO)_3L_3$$

but only under drastic condition (130–150°)[10].

Trisubstituted compounds were prepared only by displacement
reactions. Tricarbonyl(cyclohepatatriene)chromium reacted with

isonitrile in refluxing benzene[8,12], while tris(ammino)tricarbonyl-chromium reacted even at room temperature in polar solvents, such as alcohol or water (for methyl isonitrile)[14].

Trisubstituted compounds are white (CH_3NC) or yellow (aromatic isocyanides); they are all hydrophobic. They are sparingly soluble in alcohol, but soluble in different organic solvents. They are rather stable to heat and are unaffected by iodine in pyridine.

Thin-layer chromatography was successfully employed to separate mixtures of mono-, di- and trisubstituted compounds[15]: see Table 2.1.

An alternative synthesis of isocyanide complexes, not involving displacement of carbon monoxide or of other ligands, was found by Maginn[16,17]. Alkylation of the diglyme adduct of sodium penta-carbonylcyanochromate (I) with a reactive alkyl- or arylhalide in ethereal solution afforded moderate yields of the pentacarbonyl-(monoisocyanide) complex.

A brilliant extension of this method with trialkyltin (IV) chloride and with pure $Na[Cr(CO)_5CN]$ in tetrahydrofuran gave penta-carbonyl(trimethyltinisocyanide)chromium, as sublimable white crystals[18].

Acidification of $Na[Cr(CO)_5CN]$ with aqueous hydrochloric acid gave the rather unstable compound $[Cr(CO)_5(CNH)]$, purified by sublimation. Both these complexes represent a remarkable example of stabilization of a ligand otherwise not isolable. Similar compounds were prepared for molybdenum and for tungsten, and were already known in the case of iron[19].

The evidence in favour of $(HNC)Cr(CO)_5$ included a characteristic single proton n.m.r. signal ($\tau = 5.41$); moreover CO, CN and NH stretching frequencies were present. The evidence in favour of $\{(CH_3)_3SnNC\}Cr(CO)_5$ also included an n.m.r. signal corresponding to nine equivalent protons ($\tau = 9.9$–10; $J(^{119}Sn–H) = 60$ cps; $J(^{117}Sn–H) = 56$–57 cps).

Approximate force constants were calculated for the chromium, molybdenum and tungsten compounds and are reported in Table 4.1, together with constants for other $M(CO)_5L$ compounds. Comparison of the resulting force constants with those calculated by Cotton[20] for other $M(CO)_5L$ compounds indicates that the π-acceptor strength of the $(CH_3)_3ENC$ group (E = Sn, Si), of HNC and of acetonitrile are approximately equal. The great decrease in π-acceptor strength from CO to HNC indicates, according to reference 18, 'that the lone pair on the nitrogen atom is partially delocalized through structure **1** into the antibonding π^*-orbitals on the carbon atom, thus reducing the ability for HNC to accept charge from metal d orbitals '

$$\overset{\displaystyle H}{\underset{}{\diagdown}}\ \overset{\oplus}{N}\equiv C-\overset{\ominus}{M}$$

(1)

Actually there is no other evidence for a bent structure for coordinated HNC, which is a linear molecule according to its infrared spectrum in a frozen argon matrix (Table 1.1). Furthermore there is no evidence that the conclusion about the π-accepting ability of organotin isonitriles, found here to be low, has general validity. Cotton[21] found that the isocyanide ligand in the related (CH_3MNC)-$Fe(CO)_4$ (M = Ge, Si) allows back-donation, while $(CH_3)_3CNC$ does not in the analogous complex (infrared CN stretching frequency at 2132, 2135 and 2186 respectively, all in chloroform solution). It is known that isocyanides can show any intermediate behaviour between good σ-donor alone and σ-donor plus good π-acceptor. The data of Cotton and Zingales[8] on the CN and CO stretching frequencies of $Cr(CO)_3(CNR)_3$ and $Cr(CO)_5(CNR)$ suggest that the main part of back-accepting is done by the CO and not by the CNR groups (for a discussion of the available i.r. data on $(CO)_{6-n}$-$(RNC)_4M$ compounds, see under ' Derivatives of Molybdenum (o)').

Compounds with carbonyl and aromatic ligands

Compounds of this type were obtained in good yields by Strohmeier[22] by irradiation with ultraviolet light of tricarbonyl(dimethylterephthalate)chromium or of tricarbonylbenzenechromium in benzene solution containing cyclohexylisonitrile until one mole of carbon monoxide was evolved. The related compounds with mesitylene and hexamethylbenzene were not isolated in a pure state, but their infrared data could be recorded and are reported in Table 4.2.

The value of the higher, and more sensitive, carbonyl stretching frequency decreases with increasing electronic density on the chromium atom owing to the substituents on the aromatic ring. A similar decrease could be observed for the value of the CN stretching frequency and for the stability of the compounds. The span of the values of the CO stretching frequency when cyclohexylisonitrile was present (60 cm^{-1}) was practically the same as when triphenylphosphine, benzonitrile or dimethylsulphoxide were present (61, 58 and 58 cm^{-1}). The corresponding span of values for (aromatic)$Cr(CO)_2L$ was 80 cm^{-1} when L was piperidine, 78 and

3*

74 cm^{-1} when L was quinoline or pyridine, but only 40 cm^{-1} when L was CO. All these data give evidence that, at least here, the isocyanide has to be considered as a fairly good σ-donor and π-acceptor, but no difference can be appreciated from the above data alone between nitrile and isonitrile. However, comparison of the CN stretching frequency of a series of similar benzonitrile and phenylisocyanide complexes (Table 4.3) shows that the span of the complexes of the former is 34 cm^{-1}, while that in the case of the latter is 118 cm^{-1}. The wider range of values of the CN stretching frequency shows the better π-accepting ability of the isonitrile (cf. p. 27).

From the infrared evidence mentioned above and from consideration of the bond moments[13], the following scale of stability and of the related σ-donor and π-acceptor abilities was proposed by Strohmeier[22].

Stability in decreasing order	Sigma-donor ability	Pi-acceptor ability
Cr—CO (maximum)	—	Good
Cr—PR$_3$ Cr(SOMe$_2$)	Good	Medium
Cr-quinoline	Good	Small
Cr—C$_6$H$_{11}$NC	Medium	Medium
Cr—C$_6$H$_5$CN	Medium	Small
Cr—N base	Good	Absent

MOLYBDENUM

Derivatives of Molybdenum (IV)

These compounds were described by Hoelzl and Xenakis[23] in their work on the alkylation of the octacyanomolybdates (1927). Silver octacyanomolybdate was reacted with methyl iodide at mild temperature. The reaction mixture was extracted with anhydrous methanol, giving a solid residue and a solution from which a yellow crystalline substance separated. This product was very hygroscopic and had an isocyanide smell. It had an analysis corresponding to $(CH_3)_4Mo(CN)_8$ and was formulated as $Mo(CN)_4(CNCH_3)_4$, that is, as a 'methylmolybdocyanide', tetracyanotetrakis(methylisocyano)-molybdenum (IV). The solid residue was further extracted with water; the aqueous solution gave on concentration a second compound, probably derived from the above-mentioned one by hydrolysis:

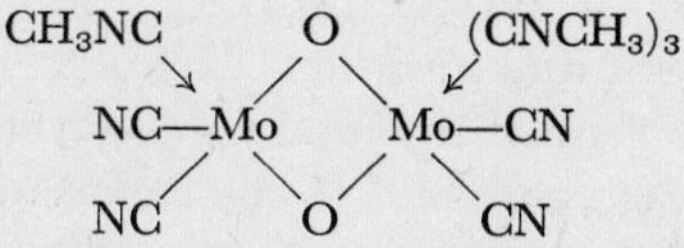

$$CH_3NC \qquad O \qquad (CNCH_3)_3$$
$$NC\!-\!Mo \qquad Mo\!-\!CN$$
$$NC \qquad O \qquad CN$$

Finally the water-insoluble residue, treated with dilute hydrochloric acid, gave a yellow solution from which other hydrolysis products were isolated, for example, those formulated as:

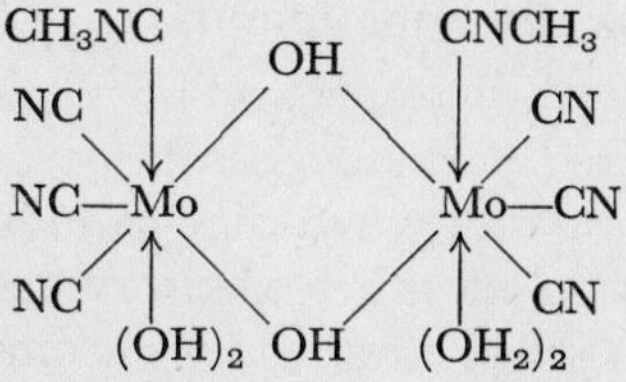

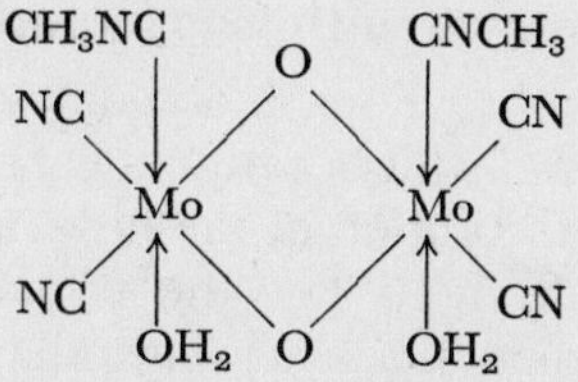

$$CH_3NC \qquad OH \qquad CNCH_3 \qquad CH_3NC \qquad O \qquad CNCH_3$$
$$NC \qquad CN \qquad NC \qquad CN$$
$$NC\!-\!Mo \qquad Mo\!-\!CN \qquad Mo \qquad Mo$$
$$NC \qquad CN \qquad NC \qquad CN$$
$$(OH)_2 \quad OH \quad (OH_2)_2 \qquad OH_2 \quad O \quad OH_2$$

Other compounds, such as $H_4[Mo(CN)_4(OH)_4].3$ $CNCH_3$, were considered addition compounds of the tetrahydroxotetracyanomolybdic (IV) acid and not true isocyanide coordination compounds.

When the methylation was carried out with $K_4[Mo(CN)_8]$ and $(CH_3)_2SO_4$, and the reaction mixture washed with water to remove CH_3SO_4K, a compound, $[Mo(CN)_4(H_2O)_2(CNCH_3)_2].4$ H_2O, was obtained which was considered to be a hydrolysis product of $Mo(CN)_4(CNCH_3)_4$.

It may be observed that these substances, though better defined than the analogous chromium (III) derivatives described by the same authors, are all rather unstable and readily hydrolyzed. These facts show that the affinity of isocyanides for Mo (IV) is still very poor.

Derivatives of Molybdenum (II)

The known complexes of molybdenum (II) contain cyclopentadienyl groups. The mustard yellow cyclopentadienylcarbonylbis(methyl-isocyanide)iodomolybdenum was obtained by refluxing overnight a mixture of $K[Mo(CN)_2(C_5H_5)(CO)_2]$ and methyl iodide in aceto-nitrile. The ether insoluble compound shows both CO and CN adsorptions in the infrared[24]. As is usual when carbonyl groups are present, the CN stretching frequencies (2185 and 2200 cm^{-1} against

2168 cm^{-1} in the free ligand) show that the isocyanide groups are very little involved in back-donation from the metal atom.

Reaction of $C_5H_5Mo(CO)_3X$ with phenylisocyanide in refluxing tetrahydrofuran gave a monosubstituted product when X was iodine and a trisubstituted product when X was chlorine. This behaviour, similar to that of the analogous carbonyl halides of iron and of manganese, was attributed to the different electronegativities of these halogens which would cause stronger back-donation in the iodide[25].

Derivatives of Molybdenum (o)

Compounds with isocyanides as the only ligands

Like chromium, molybdenum forms hexakis(aryl isocyanide)compounds[26] which can be considered formally as the products of total substitution of the hexacarbonyl although they cannot be prepared from it. For the preparation of the hexakis(arylisocyano)-molybdenum a reaction similar to that described for chromium was not possible, and one of the following methods, all giving rather poor yields, had to be adopted:

a) Reduction of an alcoholic suspension of MoO_3 with hydrazine hydroxide, in presence of an aryl isocyanide.

b) Reduction of a solution of $Mo_2O_3(S_2COC_2H_5)_4$ (an oxoethyl xanthate complex) in methylene chloride with hydrazine hydroxide in presence of an aryl isocyanide.

c) Reduction of MoO_3 to $MoCl_3$ in hydrochloric acid with magnesium powder, followed by addition of alcohol, hydrazine acetate and an aryl isocyanide.

d) Reduction of a mixture of $MoCl_3$, isocyanide and magnesium powder suspended in alcohol, by dropwise addition of glacial acetic acid. This method gave the best results. The crude products were then dissolved in methylene chloride and quickly reprecipitated by addition of anhydrous ethanol.

An alternative route to hexakis(phenyl isocyanide)molybdenum (o), by reaction of tris(dipyridyl)molybdenum with an excess of isocyanide, gave a 20% yield[4].

The hexakis(aryl isocyanide)molybdenum compounds were obtained as crystalline red powders, with golden or green reflectances, soluble in methylene chloride, chloroform and benzene, insoluble in alcohol. They are indefinitely stable in vacuum, while in the presence of air they alter within a few days; the decomposition is much more rapid in solution. Some of these compounds show a slight paramagnetism which is probably due to some impurities.

The compounds serve to initiate the polymerization of methyl methacrylate in the presence of organic halides. When compared with molybdenum hexacarbonyl in this respect, the isocyanide complexes show greater initial rates and more complicated polymerization kinetics. Free-radical formation is initiated through the abstraction of a halogen atom by the metal derivative. The paramagnetic species formed was studied through its e.s.r. spectrum; the hyperfine structure showed that it was a molybdenum compound[27]. No infrared data are available for the zerovalent molybdenum complexes.

Compounds which also contain carbonyl ligands

Details for the preparation of monophenylisocyanide-[12] or mono-anisylisocyanide-pentacarbonylmolybdenum[11] from $Mo(CO)_6$ are available. However, the preparation of all these compounds is best carried out by one of the following indirect methods:

a) Reaction of tetraethylammonium pentacarbonylchloromolybdenum (I) with isocyanide in tetrahydrofuran solution[10]: mono-, di- and tri-substituted compounds can be obtained. For details, see p. 62.

b) Displacement of the olefin in refluxing benzene from 1,5-cyclooctadiene(tetracarbonyl)molybdenum or from cycloheptatriene(tricarbonyl)molybdenum; $cis\text{-}(CNPh)_2Mo(CO)_4$[12] or $cis\text{-}(CNR)_3Mo(CO)_3$ were obtained[8,12].

c) Alkylation of $Na[Mo(CO)_5CN]$ with trimethyltin (IV) chloride. The compound had the required infrared spectrum (see Table 4.4); its n.m.r. spectrum showed a signal at $\tau = 9\cdot88$ ($J(^{119}Sn\text{—}H) = 60$ cps; $J(^{117}Sn\text{—}H) = 57$ cps). Acidification of the sodium salt afforded the unstable $(HNC)Mo(CO)_5$[18].

Direct substitution of molybdenum carbonyl with isonitrile is not a recommended method for preparing bis- and tris-isocyanide complexes. Mixtures of mono-, di- and trisubstituted complexes were obtained from the hexacarbonyl and CNPh[28], while the use of methylisocyanide gave mixtures of mono- and disubstituted compounds[29], the proportions being a function of the reaction time. The analogous reaction was reported to give only the monosubstituted products in the case of chromium and tungsten carbonyl[11]. During the reaction of molybdenum hexacarbonyl and CNPh in decalin, one mole of carbon monoxide is evolved between 90° and

110°, another mole at 125–130° and another one at ∼ 160°. However, infrared examination of the reaction mixtures showed that the solution contained all three reaction products and not only one at each temperature[28]. This fact can be explained by the observation of Murdoch that tetracarbonylbis(cyclohexylisocyanide)molybdenum disproportionates to mono- and trisubstituted product when it is heated in decalin solution at 130–150° for 1 hour[10]. Murdoch also found that mono- and disubstituted products do not react with excess isocyanide, although his study was restricted to rather mild reaction conditions (tetrahydrofuran, 48 hr, room temperature).

Mixtures of $Mo(CO)_5(CNC_6H_5)$ and $cis\text{-}Mo(CO)_4(CNC_6H_5)_2$, together with some unreacted starting material, were formed when molybdenum hexacarbonyl and phenyl isocyanate were refluxed in ethylcyclohexane. Phenylisothiocyanate afforded $Mo(CO)_3\text{-}(CNC_6H_5)_3$ in low yields. Similar reactions were also carried out for iron pentacarbonyl[30,31].

The infrared spectra in the 2000 cm^{-1} region of these compounds and of the similar ones with chromium were first examined by Cotton and Zingales[8]. They found that no remarkable change of the CN stretching frequency was observed when the spectra of pentacarbonyl(p-anisylisocyanide)molybdenum and of the free ligand were compared; similar results were also found when tris(isocyanide)-tricarbonylmetal (o) complexes were examined. Therefore, it was concluded that CO is a better π-acceptor than isocyanide. It was also remarked that alkylisocyanide is less π-accepting than arylisocyanide; moreover the presence of a CH_3, CH_3O or Cl substituent in the *para* position of the phenyl ring had little effect on the CN frequency, either in the complexes or in the free ligand.

The same conclusions were reached by Bigorgne[29], who examined the 'courbes de filiation' (Figures 4.2 and 4.3) for the series $Mo(CO)_{6-n}L_n$, where L was PMe_3, CNEt, CNPh and n was 1, 2 (*cis*) and 3 (*cis*). From the graph the following conclusions were drawn:

a) Owing to the small contribution of the π-bonding in the M–P bond, the three CO groups in $cis\text{-}Mo(CO)_3(PMe_3)_3$ can interact only between themselves through the corresponding Mo–C π-bonds. As a consequence the interaction is strong and the numerical difference between the CO frequencies is high.

b) The numerical differences between the CO frequencies in the CNPh complexes is always smaller than the corresponding

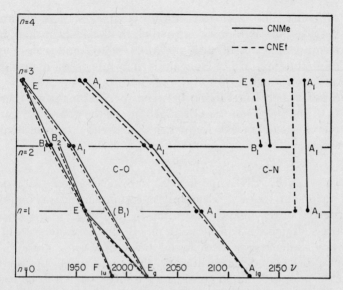

Figure 4.2 'Courbes de filiation' for $Mo(CO)_{6-n}L_n$ compounds
$(L = CNCH_3, CNC_2H_5; n = 0, 1, 2, 3)$

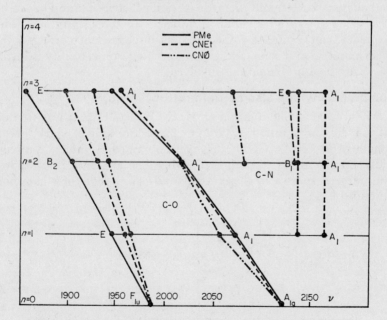

Figure 4.3 'Courbes de filiation' for $Mo(CO)_{6-n}L_n$ compounds
$(L = P(CH_3)_3, CNC_2H_5, CNC_6H_5; n = 0, 1, 2, 3)$

differences in analogous PMe$_3$ complexes. The interaction between the carbonyls is smaller in the former than in the latter complexes, because the M–(CNPh) bond is also capable of π-bonding. Ethyl isocyanide has intermediate properties, although much more on the phenyl isocyanide side.

c) Similarly, the interaction between the CNPh groups is greater than that between the CNEt groups, as the difference between the values of the CN frequencies for the first class of ligands is larger.

Force constants for the Mo(CO)$_{6-n}$L$_n$ molecules ($n = 1$, 2-*cis*, 3-*cis*; L = CNMe, CNEt and CNPh) were calculated by Horrocks[32]. For a particular series of isosymmetric compounds it was found that the ordering of the ligands according to the values of the principal CO force stretching constants parallels that obtained from raw frequency data. It was also found that the 'non rigorous' force constants calculated according to the method of Cotton[20] are similar to those calculated considering the CN stretch to be coupled to the carbonyl stretch, the only exception being the Mo(CO)$_5$-(CNR) compounds. Although the results obtained according to both methods are correct, and their use is justified, some caution has to be used when interpreting small differences in force constants. The frequency values used for the calculations were not corrected for anharmonicity and some additional and bigger uncertainty is introduced by the approximations involved.

Compounds which also contain nitrosyl groups

When an alcoholic solution of Mo(NO)$_2$(EtOH)$_2$Cl$_2$ was treated with a ligroin solution of excess phenylisocyanide, dark green crystals of Mo(NO)$_2$(CNPh)$_2$Cl$_2$ were obtained.[33] Similar diamagnetic compounds were prepared with other aromatic isocyanides. The infrared spectra of these compounds show that their common structural formula is:

TUNGSTEN

Derivatives of Tungsten (IV)

The derivatives of tungsten (IV) were prepared by Hoelzl and Zymaris (1929) by alkylation of silver octacyanotungstates (IV) with methyl iodide[34]. The various products obtained by this reaction are shown by analysis to contain tungsten, cyano groups, methyl groups and water, and it would have been possible, by analogy with the other elements of this group, to formulate them as hydrolysis products of a 'methylcyanotungstate' [tetracyanotetrakis(methylisocyano) tungstate (IV)], which can be assumed to be the primary product in the alkylation reaction:

$$Ag_4[W(CN)_8] + 4\,CH_3I \rightarrow (CH_3)_4W(CN)_8 + 4\,AgI$$

However, in order to explain why all these compounds have a strong acid reaction in aqueous solution, and why both water and isocyanide are fairly strongly bound, Hoelzl assumed them to be derivatives of $H_4[Mo(CN)_8]$, containing as ligand a product of primary hydrolysis and esterification of the isocyanide, namely, $CH_3O-C-NHCH_3$.

Thus a substance analysing as $C_8H_{16}O_2N_8W$ (2), which could have been written:

$$W[(CN)_4(CNCH_3)_4](H_2O)_2$$

was formulated by Hoelzl as:

$$H_2\left[W(CN)_6\left\{|\,C\begin{array}{c}OCH_3\\ \diagup \\ \diagdown \\ NHCH_3\end{array}\right\}_2\right]$$

Similarly, the product obtained from 2 and $AgNO_3$, which on the available analytical data could have been written:

$$Ag[W(CN)_4(OH)(CNCH_3)_3]$$

was instead formulated as:

$$Ag_2\left[\begin{array}{ccc}CH_3NC & CN & CNCH_3\\ \searrow \diagup \diagdown \swarrow\\ (NC)_4-W & & W-(CN)_4\\ \nearrow \diagdown \diagup \nwarrow\\ CH_3O-C & CN & C-OCH_3\\ | & & |\\ CH_3NC & & NHCH_3\end{array}\right]$$

and so forth.

In Hoelzl's opinion this peculiar behaviour of tungsten is due to the fact that the starting material, the silver octacyanotungstate, is actually a hydrogen silver salt of composition between Ag_3H-$[W(CN)_8]$ and $Ag_2H_2[W(CN)_8]$. Because of the acidity of the medium, the isocyanide formed by alkylation takes up a molecule of water or alcohol and gives an intermediate hydrolysis product, not stable in the free state but stable as a ligand. All this is quite possible, but in our opinion not sufficiently proved, and the suggestion that some of these compounds are derivatives of $W^{(V)}$ seems even less supported.

In any event, Hoelzl's research shows that the alkylation derivatives of $H_4[W(CN)_8]$ are undoubtedly more stable than those of $H_3[Cr(CN)_6]$ and $H_4[Mo(CN)_8]$, and that it is possible to isolate a compound of composition very near to that of the hypothetical product of primary esterification, $W(CN)_4(CNCH_3)_4$, as well as hydrolysis and condensation derivatives in which the isocyanide molecules are fairly strongly bound.

Derivatives of Tungsten (II)

The only known isocyanide complex of divalent tungsten is cyclo-pentadienyl(tricarbonyl)methylisocyanide(diiodo)tungsten. The light sensitive yellow compound was obtained by alkylation of cyclo-pentadienyl(tricarbonyl)cyanotungsten (I) with methyl iodide in acetonitrile at room temperature; it was purified by chromatography. Attempts to alkylate $K[W(CN)_2(C_5H_5)(CO)_2]$ according to the procedure used for the molybdenum analogue gave only small yields of the monoisocyanide tungsten complex[24].

Derivatives of Tungsten (0)

Compounds with isocyanides as the only ligands

The hexakis(arylisocyanide)tungsten compounds, $W(CNR)_6$, were also obtained[35], but their preparation proved very difficult and was successful only with a few aryl isocyanides, namely, phenyl, p-chlorophenyl and 2-methyl-4-chlorophenyl isocyanide. The preparation was carried out by slow addition of tungsten (VI) chloride to a mixture of isocyanide, magnesium powder, anhydrous alcohol and a few drops of glacial acetic acid. During the addition the mixture was stirred vigorously and cooled to below 0°. The precipitate thus obtained was washed thoroughly with alcohol, dissolved in benzene and chromatographed through an alumina column. On diluting the eluted solution with anhydrous alcohol, the product separated in a pure state. Yields are about 10%.

The reaction between trisdipyridyltungsten (o) and excess phenylisocyanide gave hexakis(phenylisocyanide)tungsten (o) in around 20% yield[4]. If the reaction is general, it might be a useful alternative route.

The hexakis(arylisocyanide)tungsten (o) compounds are diamagnetic crystalline substances, with red colours and green-golden reflectances. They are soluble in chloroform, methylene chloride, benzene, acetone and pyridine, insoluble in alcohol and ether. They are stable to air for a few hours.

$W(CNPh)_6$ initiates the polymerization of methyl methacrylate in the presence of organic halides, such as CCl_4. When compared with tungsten hexacarbonyl, the isocyanide compound shows greater initial rates and more complicated polymerization kinetics, although it is free from inhibition. While it was possible to detect by e.s.r. the paramagnetic species formed in the case of molybdenum compounds, in the tungsten compounds no e.s.r. signal was observed[27].

Compounds containing isocyanides with other ligands

Like chromium and molybdenum carbonyls, tungsten hexacarbonyl reacts under drastic conditions with p-anisyl isocyanide to give the monosubstituted pentacarbonyl(p-anisylisocyanide)tungsten, $W(CO)_5(CNC_7H_7O)$[11].

Reaction of tetraethylammonium pentacarbonylchlorotungstate with isocyanide at temperatures higher than 45° afforded mixtures of mono-, di- and triisocyanide complexes, as with molybdenum and chromium. However, an ionic intermediate of the reaction could be isolated at room temperature: while the mother liquor contained a mixture of all three substitution products, the orange precipitate was $[(CO)_4(C_6H_{11}NC)WCl]^-$. A similar, but less stable compound, was also isolated with phenylisocyanide. The isolation of these ionic compounds supports the mechanism proposed for the reaction (see under chromium)[10].

Alkylation of $Na[W(CO)_5CN]$ with Me_3SnCl afforded white $Me_3SnNCW(CO)_5$, while acidification of the sodium salt yielded $(HNC)W(CO)_5$. The n.m.r. spectrum of the former in benzene showed a signal at $\tau = 9.90$ ($J(^{119}Sn-H) = 60$ cps; $J(^{117}Sn-H) = 56$ cps) and that of the latter in acetone only a signal at $\tau = 4.42$. Similar chromium and molybdenum compounds were also reported[18] (see Tables 4.1, 4.2 and 4.4).

Table 4.1   Approximate force constants for some $M(CO)_5L$ compounds

Compound	CO stretching			CN stretching
	k_1	k_2	k_i	k
$(CH_3)_3SiNCMo(CO)_5$	15·13	15·92	0·18	16·98
$(CH_3)_3SnNCCr(CO)_5$	15·11	15·81	0·21	16·71
$(CH_3)_3SnNCMo(CO)_5$	15·13	15·85	0·22	16·91
$(CH_3)_3SnNCW(CO)_5$	15·06	15·74	0·22	16·89
$HNCCr(CO)_5$	15·21	16·14	0·25	17·00
$HNCMo(CO)_5$	15·32	16·06	0·26	—
$HNCW(CO)_5$	15·24	16·06	0·24	17·25
$(PCl_3)Mo(CO)_5$	16·38	16·46	0·26	—
$(Ph_3P)Mo(CO)_5$	15·57	15·99	0·31	—
$(CH_3)_3PMo(CO)_5$	15·61	15·87	0·31	—
$(C_6H_{11}NH_2)Mo(CO)_5$	14·65	15·83	0·32	—
$(n\text{-}C_3H_7)_2OMo(CO)_5$	14·65	15·90	0·35	—
$CH_3NCCr(CO)_5$	15·21	16·04	0·31	—
$CH_3CNW(CO)_5$	15·22	16·00	0·31	—

Data from ref. 18 and 20. The method of calculation employed was the same for all the compounds reported.

Table 4.2 Isocyanide compounds of chromium

Name	Formula	Colour and crystal form	M.p. °C	Note	Infrared data	Ref.
a) With isocyanides as only ligands						
Hexakis(phenyl isocyanide)chromium (o)	Cr(CNC$_6$H$_5$)$_6$	Red crystals	178·5	-327×10^{-6}[a]	CHCl$_3$:2070, 2012, 1965	3, 8
Hexakis(*p*-tolyl isocyanide)chromium (o)	Cr(CNC$_7$H$_7$)$_6$	Red crystals	152·8	-288×10^{-6}[a]	CHCl$_3$:2062, 1972, 1934	3, 8
Hexakis(*p*-anisyl isocyanide)chromium (o)	Cr(CNC$_7$H$_7$O)$_6$	Red crystals	124·4	-448×10^{-6}[a]	—	3
Hexakis(*m*-chlorophenyl isocyanide)chromium (o)	Cr(CNC$_6$H$_4$Cl)$_6$	Orange-red crystals	156	—	—	8, 3
Hexakis(*p*-chlorophenyl isocyanide)chromium (o)	Cr(CNC$_6$H$_4$Cl)$_6$	Bright red crystals	~220 (dec.)	-101×10^{-6}[a]	CHCl$_3$:2070, 2024, 1969	3, 8
Hexakis(3-chloro-2-methylphenyl isocyanide)chromium (o)	Cr(CNC$_7$H$_6$Cl)$_6$	Red crystals	192·5	-541×10^{-6}[a]	—	3
Hexakis(4-chloro-2-methylphenyl isocyanide)chromium (o)	Cr(CNC$_7$H$_6$Cl)$_6$	Red crystals with golden reflectances	172	—	—	3
Hexakis(2,4-dimethyl isocyanide)chromium (o)	Cr(CNC$_8$H$_9$)$_6$	Red crystals	—	—	—	3
Hexakis(2,5-dichlorophenyl isocyanide)chromium (o)	Cr(CNC$_6$H$_3$Cl$_2$)$_6$	Red crystals with golden reflectances	166	-127×10^{-6}[a]	—	3
Hexakis(allyl isocyanide)chromium (o)	Cr(CNC$_2$H$_3$)$_6$	Orange crystals	—	—	—	36
b) With carbonyl groups[d]						
Pentacarbonyl(trimethylsilyl isocyanide)chromium (o)	Cr(CO)$_5$(CNC$_3$H$_9$Sn)	White crystals	148–150 subl. 135/0·1[b,e]		mull:2101w(CN);2035m, 1928w, sh; 1953vs; 2950, 2980vvw	18
Pentacarbonyl(hydrogen isocyanide)chromium (o)	Cr(CO)$_5$(CNH)	White crystals	114–116 subl. 60–90/0·1[c,e] dec.		mull:2115vw(CN); 2066vw, 1934w, sh; 1968s; 3360s (NH)	18, 37
Pentacarbonyl(*p*-anisyl isocyanide)chromium (o)	Cr(CO)$_5$(CNC$_7$H$_7$O)	Colourless needles	107–108	—	—	11
Pentacarbonyl(phenyl isocyanide)chromium (o)	Cr(CO)$_5$(CNC$_6$H$_5$)	Pale yellow	65–66 55–56	subl. 40–60/0·1	CHCl$_3$:2125(CN); 2040, 1963	10 12
Pentacarbonyl(cyclohexyl isocyanide)chromium (o)	Cr(CO)$_5$(CNC$_6$H$_{11}$)	Colourless	49	subl. 40–60/0·1; dipole moment	—	12, 13

[a] Magnetic susceptibility at 18°c (χ_m).

[b] Ultraviolet spectrum in CH$_2$Cl$_2$: maximum at 238 mμ (61,000).

[c] Ultraviolet spectrum in CH$_2$Cl$_2$:maximum at 235 mμ (45,000).

[d] [(HNC)Cr(CO)$_5$]$_2$·ROCH$_2$CH$_2$OR (R = CH$_3$, C$_2$H$_5$, n-C$_3$H$_7$) were reported (16), but their formulation was changed to oxonium salt (18).

[e] ^{1}H n.m.r. spectrum reported in the text.

Table 4.2 (*continued*)

Name	Formula	Colour and crystal form	M.p. °C	Note	Infrared data	Ref.
Pentacarbonyl(diphenylmethyl isocyanide)-chromium (o)	$Cr(CO)_5(CNC_{13}H_{11})$	—	52–53	—	—	16
Pentacarbonyl(triphenylmethyl isocyanide)chromium (o)	$Cr(CO)_5(CNC_{19}H_{15})$	—	135–136	—	—	16
Pentacarbonyl(benzoyl isocyanide)-chromium (o)	$Cr(CO)_5(CNC_7H_5O)$	—	85–86	—	—	17
Pentacarbonyl(isobutyryl isocyanide)-chromium (o)	$Cr(CO)_5(CNC_4H_9)$	—	55–57	—	—	17
cis-Tetracarbonylbis(phenyl isocyanide)-chromium (o)	$Cr(CO)_4(CNC_6H_5)_2$	Pale yellow	86–87	sublimable high vacuum	$C_{16}H_{34}$:2015, 1956, 1946; 2065, 2130(CO)	10
trans-Tetracarbonylbis(cyclohexyl isocyanide)-chromium (o)	$Cr(CO)_4(CNC_6H_{11})_2$	—	87–88	dipole moment	—	12
cis-Tetracarbonylbis(cyclohexyl isocyanide)-chromium (o)	$Cr(CO)_4(CNC_6H_{11})_2$	Pale yellow	95–96	—	—	13
Tricarbonyltris(methyl isocyanide)-chromium (o)	$Cr(CO)_3(CNCH_3)_3$	White crystals	157 dec.	—	CH_2Cl_2:2185, 2147; 1942, 1860(CO)	8, 14
cis-Tricarbonyltris(phenyl isocyanide)-chromium (o)	$Cr(CO)_3(CNC_6H_5)_3$	Yellow	108–109	—	$CHCl_3$:2125, 2055; 1953, 1915 (CO)	10, 12, 14
Tricarbonyltris(p-tolyl isocyanide)-chromium (o)	$Cr(CO)_3(CNC_7H_7)_3$	Yellow crystals	145	—	$CHCl_3$:2150, 2085, 2047sh; 1950, 1902 (CO)	8
cis-Tricarbonyltris(p-tolyl isocyanide)-chromium (o)	$Cr(CO)_3(CNC_7H_{11})_3$	Yellow	97	—	—	10
Tricarbonyltris(p-anisyl isocyanide)-chromium (o)	$Cr(CO)_3(CNC_7H_7O)_3$	Yellow	—	—	—	14
c) With carbonyl and aromatic groups						
Dicarbonylbenzene(cyclohexyl isocyanide)-chromium (o)	$Cr(CO)_2(C_6H_6)(CNC_6H_{11})$	Yellow	>90 dec.	—	2083 (CN), 1912 (CO)[f]	22
Dicarbonyl(dimethylterephthalate)-(cyclohexyl isocyanide)chromium (o)	$Cr(CO)_2(C_{10}H_{10}O_4)$-$(CNC_6H_{11})$	Ruby-red	126	dipole moment[g]	2123 (CN), 1940 (CO)[f]	13, 22
Dicarbonylmesitylene(cyclohexyl isocyanide)chromium (o)	$Cr(CO)_2(C_9H_{12})(CNC_6H_{11})$	Not isolated in pure state	—	—	2044 (CN), 1902 (CO)[f]	22
Dicarbonyl(hexamethylbenzene)cyclohexyl isocyanide)chromium (o)	$Cr(CO)_2(C_{12}H_{18})(CNC_6H_{11})$	Not isolated in pure state	—	—	2005 (CN), 1880 (CO)[f]	22

[f] Only the higher CO stretching frequency was reported.

[g] Aromatic signals at 328 cps. from $(CH_3)_4Si$, benzene being at 436 cps.

Table 4.3   CN stretching frequency for some benzonitrile and phenyl isocyanide complexes[22]

Compound	L = C_6H_5CN	L = C_6H_5NC
Free ligand (L)	2227	2158
(Diethylterephthalate) $Cr(CO)_2(L)$	2222	2123
(Benzene)$Cr(CO)_2(L)$	2212	2083
(Mesitylene)$Cr(CO)_2(L)$	2203	2044
(Hexamethylbenzene)$Cr(CO)_2(L)$	2188	2005

Table 4.4 Isocyanide compounds of molybdenum

Name	Formula	Colour and crystal form	M.p. °C	Note	Infrared data	Ref.
a) With isocyanides as only ligands						
Hexakis(phenyl isocyanide)-molybdenum (o)	$Mo(CNC_6H_5)_6$	Red needles with green reflectances	—	207×10^{-6a}	—	4, 26
Hexakis(p-tolyl isocyanide)-molybdenum (o)	$Mo(CNC_7H_7)_6$	Orange leaflets	—	—	—	26
Hexakis(m-chlorophenyl isocyano)-molybdenum (o)	$Mo(CNC_6H_4Cl)_6$	Yellow-orange crystals	—	—	—	26
Hexakis(4-chloro-2-methylphenyl isocyanide)molybdenum (o)	$Mo(CNC_7H_6Cl)_6$	Yellow-orange crystals	—	156×10^{-6a}	—	26
Hexakis(6-chloro-2-methylphenyl isocyanide)molybdenum (o)	$Mo(CNC_7H_6Cl)_6$	Brick-red crystals	—	156×10^{-6a}	—	26
Hexakis(2,4-dichlorophenyl isocyanide)-molybdenum (o)	$Mo(CNC_6H_3Cl_2)_6$	Yellow-orange crystals	—	—	—	26
b) With carbonyl groups						
Pentacarbonyl(cyclohexyl isocyanide)-molybdenum (o)	$Mo(CO)_5(CNC_6H_{11})$	—	—	dipole moment $5 \cdot 70D(C_6H_{12})$	—	13
Pentacarbonyl[(p-anisyl isocyanide)-molybdenum (o)	$Mo(CO)_5(CNC_7H_7O)$	Colourless crystals	105–106	—	$CHCl_3$:2145 (CN); 2062, 1953	8, 11
Pentacarbonyl(phenyl isocyanide)-molybdenum (o)	$Mo(CO)_5(CNC_6H_5)$	—	66–67, 74	—	$CHCl_3$:2135 (CN); 2050, 1965	10, 12, 30
Pentacarbonyl(methyl isocyanide)-molybdenum (o)	$Mo(CO)_5(CNCH_3)$	—	—	—	$C_{16}H_{34}$:2178 (CN); 2071, 1960	29
Pentacarbonyl(ethyl isocyanide)-molybdenum (o)	$Mo(CO)_5(CNC_6H_{11})$	Colourless	86	—	—	10
cis-Tetracarbonylbis(methyl isocyanide)-molybdenum (o)	$Mo(CO)_4(CNCH_3)_2$	—	—	—	$C_{16}H_{34}$:2176, 2140 (CN); 2022, 1943, 1931, 1923	29
cis-Tetracarbonylbis(ethyl isocyanide)-molybdenum (o)	$Mo(CO)_4(CNC_2H_5)_2$	—	—	—	$C_{16}H_{34}$:2165, 2131 (CN); 2018, 1941, 1930, 1921	29
cis-Tetracarbonylbis(cyclohexyl isocyanide)-molybdenum (o)	$Mo(CO)_4(CNC_6H_{11})_2$	Pale yellow	108	—	4 CO stretchings	10

Compound	Formula	Colour	M.p. (°C)	Sublimation	Infrared/spectroscopic data (cm⁻¹)	References
cis-Tetracarbonyl(phenyl isocyanide)molybdenum (o)	$Mo(CO)_4(CNC_6H_5)_2$	Colourless	106–107	sublimable in high vacuum	$C_{16}H_{34}$:2130, 2070; 2020, 1953, 1943 4 CO stretchings	8, 12, 30
cis-Tricarbonyltris(methyl isocyanide)molybdenum	$Mo(CO)_3(CNCH_3)_3$	Colourless	—	—	$C_{16}H_{34}$:2174, 2133 (CN); 1957, 1896	10
cis-Tricarbonyltris(ethyl isocyanide)molybdenum (o)	$Mo(CO)_3(CNC_2H_5)_3$	Colourless	—	—	$C_{16}H_{34}$:2160, 2122 (CN); 1952, 1895	29
cis-Tricarbonyltris(cyclohexyl isocyanide)molybdenum (o)	$Mo(CO)_3(CNC_6H_{11})_3$	Yellow	—	—	—	29
cis-Tricarbonyltris(phenyl isocyanide)molybdenum (o)	$Mo(CO)_3(CNC_6H_5)_3$	Colourless	144–145	—	$CHCl_3$:2130, 2065 (CN); 1953, 1915	10
Tricarbonyltri(p-tolyl isocyanide)molybdenum (o)	$Mo(CO)_3(CNC_7H_7)_3$	Yellow	—	—	$CHCl_3$:2142, 2083, 2040sh (CN); 1950, 1894	10, 12, 30
Pentacarbonyl(hydrogen isocyanide)molybdenum (o)	$Mo(CO)_5(CNH)$	White	Unstable	subl. 70–80/0.1ᵇ	C_6H_{12}:2067vw, 1938vw, 1962m (CO); 3350vw (NH)	8
Pentacarbonyl(trimethylstannyl isocyanide)molybdenum (o)	$Mo(CO)_5(CNC_3H_9Sn)$	White	152–153	subl. 130–150/0.1 τ 9·98 (C_6H_6)ᶜ	C_6H_{12}:2112w (CN); 2033m, 1932w, 1963vs; 2925vvw (CH,KBr)	18
e) With π-cyclopentadienyl- or cyano- groups						
Cyclopentadienyldicarbonyl(phenyl isocyanide)iodomolybdenum (II)	$MoI(C_5H_5)(CO)_2(CNC_6H_5)$	Red	75	—	C_6H_{12}:2108w (CN); 2042m, 1928m, sh, 1954vs (CO)	18
Cyclopentadienyltris(phenyl isocyanide)iodomolybdenum (II)	$MoI(C_5H_5)(CNC_6H_5)_3$	Red	180 dec.	—	CCl_4:2141s, 2070m, 2004s, 1942s	25
Cyclopentadienylcarbonylbis(methyl isocyanide)iodomolybdenum (II)	$MoI(C_5H_5)(CO)(CNCH_3)$	Mustard yellow	180–182	—	KCl:2169m, 2096s; 1945, 2000 (CO); 2185, 2200 (CN)	24
d) With nitrosyl groups						
Dinitrosylbis(phenyl isocyanide)dichloromolybdenum (o)	$MoCl_2(NO)_2(CNC_6H_5)_2$	Dark green	182	—	CH_2Cl_2:1804vs, 1706vs; 2208vs, 2160w (CN)	33
Dinitrosylbis(p-tolyl isocyanide)dichloromolybdenum (o)	$MoCl_2(NO)_2(CNC_7H_7)_2$	Dark green	190	—	CH_2Cl_2:1805vs, 1705vs; 2200vs, 2160w (CN)	33
Dinitrosylbis(p-benzyl isocyanide)dichloromolybdenum (o)	$MoCl_2(NO)_2(CNC_7H_7)_2$	Yellow-green	142	—	CH_2Cl_2:1808s, 1692vs; 2280m, 2240w	33

ᵃ Magnetic susceptibility of the solid compound, χ_M, at 20°C.
ᵇ Ultraviolet spectrum in CH_2Cl_2 solution: 233 mμ (132,000) and 288 mμ (21,000).
ᶜ Ultraviolet spectrum in CH_2Cl_2 solution: 238 mμ (124,000).

Table 4.5 Isocyanide compounds of tungsten

Name	Formula	Colour and crystal form	M.p. °C	Note	Infrared data	Ref.
Hexakis(phenyl isocyanide)tungsten (o)	$W(CNC_6H_5)_6$	Dark red prisms	120–130	186×10^{-6}[a]	—	4, 35
Hexakis(p-chlorophenyl isocyanide)-tungsten (o)	$W(CNC_6H_4Cl)_6$	Red prisms with gold-green reflectances	—	240×10^{-6}[a]	—	35
Hexakis(3-chloro-2-methylphenyl isocyanide)tungsten (o)	$W(CNC_7H_6Cl)_6$	Red prisms with green reflectances	205–207	203×10^{-6}[a]	—	35
Pentacarbonyl(cyclohexyl isocyanide)-tungsten (o)	$W(CO)_5(CNC_6H_{11})$	Colourless	76	subl. 40–60°/0·1	—	10
Pentacarbonyl(phenyl isocyanide)-tungsten (o)	$W(CO)_5(CNC_6H_5)$	Pale yellow	80	subl. 40–60°/0·1	—	10
Pentacarbonyl(β-anisyl isocyanide)-tungsten (o)	$W(CO)_5(CNC_7H_7O)$	Colourless needles	121·5	—	—	11
Pentacarbonyl(hydrogen isocyanide)-tungsten (o)	$W(CO)_5(NCH)$	White	>105 dec.	subl. 70–90°/0·1 τ4·42 (acetone)[b]	KBr:2130w (CN), 3300s	18
Pentacarbonyl(trimethylstannyl isocyanide)tungsten (o)	$W(CO)_5(CNC_3H_9Sn)$	White	177–178	subl. 130/0·1 τ4·42 (acetone)[c]	C6H12:2062vw, 1934w, 1964s C6H12:2107w (CN), 2035m, 1923w, sh, 1947vs	37 18
cis-Tetracarbonylbis(cyclohexyl isocyanide)-tungsten (o)	$W(CO)_4(CNC_6H_{11})_2$	Pale yellow	107	—	4 CO stretchings	10
cis-Tetracarbonylbis(phenyl isocyanide)-tungsten (o)	$W(CO)_4(CNC_6H_5)_2$	Pale yellow	116	—	4 CO stretchings	10
cis-Tricarbonyltris(cyclohexyl isocyanide)-tungsten (o)	$W(CO)_3(CNC_6H_{11})_3$	Yellow	121	—	—	10
cis-Tricarbonyltris(phenyl isocyanide)-tungsten (o)	$W(CO)_3(CNC_6H_{11})_3$	Yellow	145–146	—	—	10
Tetraethylammonium cis-tetracarbonyl-(phenyl isocyanide)chlorotungstato (o)	$[C_8H_{20}N][WCl(CO)_4(CNC_6H_5)]$	Orange	88	—	CH2Cl2:2112 (CN); 1996s, 1891vs, 1875sh, 1937s	10
Tetraethylammonium tetracarbonyl(cyclohexyl isocyanide)chloro-tungstato (o)	$[C_8H_{20}N][WCl(CO)_4(CNC_6H_{11})]$	Orange	67–68	—	CH2Cl2:2146 (CN); 1999m, 1885vs, 1864, 1806s	10
Tetraethylammonium tricarbonylbis-(phenyl isocyanide)chlorotungstato (o)	$[C_8H_{20}N][WCl(CO)_3(CNC_6H_5)_2]$	Deep-red orange	134–135 dec.	unstable in solution	Nujol:2120, 2075 (CN); 1912vs, 1860m, 1780s	10
Cyclopentadienyltricarbonyl(methyl isocyanide)tungsten (II) iodide	$[W(C_5H_5)(CO)_3(CNCH_3)]I$	Yellow	153 change	light-sensitive	1985vs, 2080s (CO), 2230m (CN)	24

[a] Magnetic susceptibility at room temperature.
[b] Ultraviolet spectrum in CH2Cl2:233 mμ (147,000) and 290 mμ (11,700).
[c] Ultraviolet spectrum in CH2Cl2:234 mμ (125,000).

REFERENCES

1. F. Hoelzl and F. Viditz, *Monatsh.*, **49**, 241 (1928).
2. L. Malatesta and A. Sacco, *Atti Accad. naz. Lincei, Rend. Classe Sci. fis. mat. nat.*, *VIII*, **13**, 264 (1952).
3. L. Malatesta, A. Sacco and S. Ghielmi, *Gazz. Chim. Ital.*, **82**, 516 (1952).
4. S. Herzog and E. Gutsche, *Z. Chem.*, **3**, 393 (1963).
5. *British Patent*, 854,615; *Chem. Abs.*, **55**, 10798b (1961).
6. *Italian Patent*, 599,661; *Chem. Abs.*, **55**, 18193c (1961).
7. G. Cetini and O. Gambino, *Ann. Chim. (Italy)*, **53**, 236 (1963).
8. F. A. Cotton and F. Zingales, *J. Am. Chem. Soc.*, **83**, 351 (1961).
9. F. A. Cotton, T. G. Dunne and J. S. Wood, *Inorg. Chem.*, **4**, 318 (1965).
10. H. D. Murdoch and R. Henzi, *J. Organomet. Chem.*, **5**, 166 (1966).
11. W. Hieber and D. Von Pigeno, *Chem. Ber.*, **89**, 616 (1956).
12. G. Cetini, A. Gambino and M. Castiglioni, *Atti R. Accad. Sci. Torino. Classe Sci. fis. mat.*, **97**, 1131 (1963).
13. W. Strohmeier and H. Hellmann, *Ber. Bunsenges. Physik. Chem.*, **68**, 481 (1964).
14. W. Hieber, W. Abeck and H. K. Platzer, *Z. anorg. Chem.*, **280**, 252 (1955).
15. G. Cetini, personal communication (Rome, April 1967).
16. *U.S. Patent*, 3,136,799; *Chem. Abs.*, **61**, 7044 d (1964).
17. *U.S. Patent*, 3,136,797; *Chem. Abs.*, **61**, 7044 f (1964).
18. R. B. King, *Inorg. Chem.*, **6**, 25 (1967).
19. D. Seyferth and N. Kahlen, *J. Am. Chem. Soc.*, **82**, 1080 (1960).
20. F. A. Cotton, *Inorg. Chem.*, **3**, 702 (1964).
21. F. A. Cotton and R. V. Parish, *J. Chem. Soc.*, **1960**, 1440.
22. W. Strohmeier and H. Hellmann, *Chem. Ber.*, **97**, 1877 (1964).
23. F. Hoelzl and G. Is. Xenakis, *Monatsh.*, **48**, 689 (1927).
24. C. E. Coffey, *J. Inorg. Nucl. Chem.*, **25**, 179 (1963).
25. K. K. Joshi, P. L. Pauson and W. H. Stubbs, *J. Organomet. Chem.*, **1**, 51 (1963).
26. L. Malatesta, A. Sacco and M. Gabaglio. *Gazz. Chim. Ital.*, **82**, 548 (1952).
27. C. H. Bamford, G. G. Eastmond and K. Hargreaves, *Nature*, **205**, 385 (1965).
28. M. Bigorgne and L. Rassat, *Bull. Soc. chim. France*, **1963**, 295.
29. M. Bigorgne and A. Bouquet, *J. Organomet. Chem.*, **1**, 101 (1963).
30. T. A. Manuel, *Inorg. Chem.*, **3**, 1703 (1964).
31. H. Ulrich, B. Tucker and A. A. R. Sayigh, *Tetrahedron Letters*, **1967**, 1731.
32. G. R. Van Hecke and W. DeW. Horrocks, Jr., *Inorg. Chem.*, **5**, 1960 (1966).
33. F. Canziani, U. Sartorelli and F. Cariati, *Ann. Chim.*, **54**, 1354 (1964).
34. F. Hoelzl and N. Zymaris, *Monatsh.* **49**, 241 (1928).
35. L. Malatesta and A. Sacco, *Ann. Chim. (Italy)*, **43**, 622 (1953).
36. D. S. Matteson and R. A. Bailey, *Chem. and Ind.*, **1967**, 191.
37. J. F. Guttenberger, *Abstracts*, 3rd International Symposium on Organometallic Chemistry, Munich (1967), p. 96.

5 ISOCYANIDE COMPLEXES OF GROUP VII ELEMENTS

Only manganese and rhenium derivatives are known, the latter being far less numerous and not always well documented. Zerovalent derivatives are known only in the case of manganese, while the $+1$ oxidation state is the most stable in both elements.

Compounds with metal–metal bond are probably known for both elements [dimeric $ReCl_3.CNR$ and $Mn_2(CO)_8(CNPh)_2$] but confirmation is still lacking.

MANGANESE

Manganese (ii) salts, as well as the coordination compounds of Mn (ii) and Mn (iii), do not show any tendency to react with isocyanides under the most varied conditions. This is probably the reason why no isocyanide derivatives of manganese were known until relatively recently.

Derivatives of manganese (II)

The $+2$ oxidation state is usual for manganese in all its simple and in most of its complex salts. Yet the isocyanide derivatives of manganese (II)[1,2], in their general features as well as in their way of preparation, constitute a class of compounds quite apart from the other known complexes of divalent manganese.

Ethyl and t-butyl isocyanide complexes $[(RNC)_6Mn]^{2+}$ were prepared by oxidation with nitric acid of the corresponding manganese (I) complexes; they were precipitated as white crystals by addition to an aqueous solution of sodium hexafluorophosphate. Vinyl and phenyl isocyanide complexes were prepared as the tetrabromocadmiates by nitric acid oxidation of a solution of a $[(RNC)_6-Mn]^+$ complex in the presence of cadmium bromide. Analogous derivatives of other aromatic isocyanides were obtained by anodic oxidation or by bromine oxidation in alcoholic solution. The perchlorate was obtained by oxidation with potassium permanganate in the presence of perchloric acid. The nitrate was obtained by oxidation of the univalent nitrate with the calculated amount of the concentrated nitric acid in glacial acetic acid; it is readily soluble in alcohol and is a very suitable intermediate for the preparation of other salts, such as the tetraiodomercurate or the picrate.

While the hexa(alkyl isocyanide)manganese (II) cations are colourless, $[Mn(CNCH{=}CH_2)_6]CdBr_4$ is dark red, and the salts of hexakis(aryl isocyanide)manganese (II) cations are blue-violet crystalline substances. They are soluble in methylene chloride, chloroform, acetone and glacial acetic acid, sparingly soluble in benzene and alcohol. In the solid state, and in solution in chloroform or glacial acetic acid, they are stable for several months. They are not affected by strong mineral acid, but decompose immediately in presence of alkali, probably according to the equation:

$$13\,[Mn(CNR)_6]^{2+} + 14\,OH^- \rightarrow$$
$$12\,[Mn(CNR)_6]^+ + 6\,RNCO + Mn(OH)_2 + 6\,H_2O$$

An analogous reduction takes place in the presence of free isocyanide. Therefore, since the solutions of the hexakis(aryl isocyanide)-manganese (II) salts are stable for quite a long time, it may be inferred that the stability constant of the cation $[Mn(CNR)_6]^{2+}$ is very high.

All the reported magnetic moments[1,2] indicate only one unpaired electron. Although the value of the crystal-field splitting in an octahedral d^5 complex (Δ_0) required to produce a t_{2g}^5 configuration, instead of the prevalent $t_{2g}^3\, e_{2g}^2$ configuration, is quite high, this is possible with strong ligands, which can increase Δ_0 by means of π-bonding. This is indeed the case with $[Mn(CNR)_6]^{2+}$, $[Mn(CN)_6]^{4-}$ and $[Mn(CN)_5NO]^{3-}$.

Infrared data are available for these complexes[2,3]; they are discussed together with those concerning Mn^I derivatives.

Derivatives of manganese (I)

Compounds with isocyanides as the only ligands

Sacco observed[4] that the anhydrous manganese (II) iodide behaves differently from the other manganous salts. In alcoholic solution it reacts with alkyl and aryl isocyanides according to the equation:

$$2\,MnI_2 + 12\,CNR \rightarrow [Mn(CNR)_6]I + [Mn(CNR)_6]I_3$$

This reaction is not a disproportionation of the type Mn (II) → Mn (I) + Mn (III), as it might appear at first, because the compound $[Mn(CNR)_6]I_3$ is not a derivative of manganese (III) but a triiodide of hexaisocyanidemanganese (I). This formulation agrees with the following facts: (a) the compound $[Mn(CNR)_6]I_3$ is diamagnetic, while a hexacoordinated cation of Mn (III) would be expected to be paramagnetic; (b) in nitrobenzene solution, its electrical conductivity has the standard value for a strong uni–univalent electrolyte; and (c) it can be reduced to the corresponding iodide under the same mild conditions required for the reduction of iodine to iodide ion (e.g. with thiosulphate). On the other hand, the oxidation of $[Mn(CNR)_6]^+$ with strong oxidizing agents leads to the corresponding Mn (II) compound, but on no account can the trivalent derivatives be obtained.

The separation of the iodide and triiodide from the reaction mixture is usually easy because of their different solubilities in alcohol, the iodide being much more soluble.

In the case of methyl isocyanide, however, the iodide is so soluble that it would be very difficult to obtain it in a pure state from the original alcoholic solution. The hexakis(methyl isocyanide)manganese (I) iodide was best prepared in the following way; by addition of iodine to the reaction mixture, all the iodide was converted into the less soluble triiodide, which was separated, purified and then quantitatively reconverted into the iodide by shaking a chloroform solution with aqueous sodium thiosulphate.

The hexa(isocyanide)manganese (I) iodide compounds, on reaction with silver oxide in aqueous alcoholic suspension or by treatment with an ion-exchange resin[5] give the corresponding hydroxides, $[Mn(CNR)_6]OH$. These are stable crystalline substances, with strong alkaline character. Chloroform solutions of the hydroxides extract Cl^-, Br^-, I^-, SCN^-, CrO_4^-, MoO_4^{2-} and WO_4^{2-} from their aqueous solutions[5].

The fact that the hydroxides of hexa(isocyanide)manganese (I) ions may be transformed into stable crystalline bicarbonates, $[Mn(CNR)_6]HCO_3$, shows that their base strengths are comparable with those of the alkali hydroxides. In fact, only the alkali metals form bicarbonates that are stable in the solid state.

From the iodide by an exchange reaction or from the hydroxide with the corresponding acid, many salts of hexa(isocyanide)-manganese (I) ions were prepared[6], namely, chlorides, bromides, chlorates, perchlorates, hydrogen carbonates, carbonates, tetra-fluoroborates, tetraphenylborates and hexafluorophosphates. Nitrates were obtained from the iodide by use of an anion-exchange column[2]. Except when the anion itself is coloured, these salts are colourless when R is an alkyl (methyl, ethyl, cyclohexyl, benzyl) and yellow when R is an aryl (phenyl, p-tolyl, p-anisyl-, p-chloro-phenyl). They are soluble in methylene chloride, chloroform and nitrobenzene, slightly soluble in benzene. The solubility in alcohol varies greatly, depending on the isocyanide and on the anion. They are all diamagnetic, as expected for hexacoordinated complexes of Mn^I with strong ligands, and in nitrobenzene solution behave as strong uni–univalent electrolytes. The tetraphenylborate of hexakis(aryl isocyanide)manganese (I), which is not dissociated in anhydrous benzene, has an extraordinarily high dipole moment (about 22 D)[7].

The salts of hexa(isocyanide)manganese (I) are indefinitely stable to air both in the solid state and in solution, and melt, generally without decomposition, in a high temperature range (150–250°). This quite unusual thermal stability shows that the coordination of isocyanides to manganese (I) results in the stabilization not only of the unusual valence state for the metal, but also of isocyanides with respect to oxidation, polymerization and rearrangement to cyanides.

It may be noticed that Cr^0, Mn^I and Fe^{II} form a series of iso-electronic hexacoordinated isocyanide compounds—$Cr(CNR)_6$,

$[Mn(CNR)_6]^+$ and $[Fe(CNR)_6]^{2+}$—in which, as in the analogous series—$[Co(CNR)_5]^+$, $Ni(CNR)_4$ and $[Cu(CNR)_4]^+$—the metal atom has reached the e.a.n. (effective atomic number) of krypton.

Comparable hexa(isonitrile)manganese (I) and (II) derivatives are available and the CN stretching frequencies of $[Mn(p\text{-}CH_3C_6H_4NC)_6]^{n+}$ ($n = 1, 2$) have been compared[3]. The value for the Mn^I compound (2090 cm^{-1} in chloroform) is lower than the value recorded for the free isonitrile (2136 cm^{-1}) and this is in turn lower than the value found for the Mn^{II} derivatives (2161 cm^{-1}, nujol). This is due to the greater electrostatic driving force for donation in the Mn^{II} than in the Mn^I cation. When the CN stretching bands in the p-tolyl and methyl isocyanide derivatives of manganese (I) are compared (2090 and 2129 cm^{-1} respectively), the lowering of the values in comparison with those of the free ligands is in agreement with the better π-acceptor character of the aromatic isocyanides, as already seen, for example, in the $Mo(CO)_3(CNR)_3$ compounds.

Compounds containing both isocyanides and other ligands

They were obtained by reaction of a manganese (I) carbonyl derivative with an isonitrile. Irradiation of a pentane solution of cyclopentadienyltricarbonylmanganese (I) and cyclohexyl isonitrile gave a low yield of $C_5H_5Mn(CO)_2(CNC_6H_{11})$ after 2–3 hours[8]. A better yield was obtained when cyclohexyl isocyanide displaced pyridine from $C_5H_5Mn(CO)_2Py$ (ethanol, 70°, 5 m)[9].

From a comparison of the carbonyl stretching frequencies of the compound with those of other compounds having different donor molecules in place of cyclohexyl isocyanide, it was found[9] that dialkyl sulphite and sulphur dioxide are better back-acceptors than isocyanides, and that the latter allows more extensive back-donation than do Ph_3P, Ph_3As, Ph_3Sb and thioethers.

Direct substitution of all the carbonyl groups with isocyanide has not been described. However, stable cyclopentadienyltris-(phenyl isocyanide)manganese (I) is known; it was obtained in 20% yield by addition of a solution of hexakis(phenyl isocyanide)manganese (I) iodide in dimethylformamide to sodium cyclopentadienide in tetrahydrofuran[10].

The extent of carbon monoxide substitution by an isonitrile is a function of the solvent[11]. Bromopentacarbonylmanganese was reported to yield mono-[10] and bis-[12] isocyanide derivatives in dichlorobenzene or ethanol as a solvent. While a similar bis-isocyanide derivative was obtained[11] in the same reaction conditions, in diglyme at 100° the reaction proceeded to the next stage, yielding bromodi-carbonyltris(phenylisocyanide)manganese (I). The influence and the role of the solvent was shown by the formation of three moles of CO per mole of metal carbonyl when the latter was heated with diglyme alone. The use of a more basic solvent, such as tetrahydro-furan, afforded $[MnBr(CO)(CNPh)_4]$ accompanied by $[MnBr(CNPh)_5]$; the latter was also obtained by reaction of the former with more isocyanide. The reactivities of $MnX(CO)_5$ molecules with X = Cl, I are different from that of the bromide. The decreasing electronegativity from Cl to I will lead to the strongest metal–carbon bonding here. This is in agreement with the measured carbonyl stretching frequencies and with the chemical reactivity towards phenyl isocyanide, as can be seen below.

$$MnX(CO)_5 \begin{cases} \xrightarrow{X = Cl} [Mn(CNPh)_6]Cl \\ \xrightarrow{X = Br} MnBr(CO)(CNPh)_4 + MnBr(CNPh)_5 \\ \xrightarrow{X = I} MnI(CO)(CNPh)_4 \end{cases}$$

Infrared data, in different media, are available for identification of the compounds.

The kinetics of the reaction between $Mn(CO)_5Br$ and ethyl isocyanide in chlorobenzene at 40°C have been studied; a solvent effect is present[13].

Derivatives of manganese (0)

Only two zerovalent manganese complexes with isocyanides are known: $Mn_2(CO)_9(CNPh)$ and $Mn_2(CO)_8(CNPh)_2$. They were isolated in low yields from the reaction of methyl- or phenylpenta-carbonylmanganese and the ligand in tetrahydrofuran. The fate of the methyl and phenyl groups in the reactions was not determined. The infrared spectra do not give any evidence for bridging carbonyl or isocyanide groups[11].

RHENIUM

As with manganese the compounds of Re^I are either carbonyl halides or hexakis(isonitrile)compounds. Infrared and other physical data are still lacking.

The first product of the reaction between rhenium triiodide or trichloride and an isonitrile analyses as a 1:1 addition compound and is reported to be dimeric. Upon further treatment with pure

4+I.C.M.

isonitrile at 150°, this undergoes an exothermic reaction, yielding $Re(CNR)_6I_3$, together with a small amount of $Re(CNR)_6I$, separated by fractional crystallization. The former compound has to be considered as a triiodide of Re^I and not as an iodide of a hexacoordinate Re^{III}. Indeed, by reaction of the triiodide or of the iodide with sodium tetraphenylborate, the same product was obtained, namely $[Re(CNR)_6]$ $[B(C_6H_5)_4]$. The iodide is best prepared by reduction of the triiodide with alcoholic $NaBH_4$. This was the starting material to prepare a number of other salts, including the nitrate and the perchlorate, by exchange reactions. All these salts are well-crystallized substances, soluble in polar solvents, stable to air both in the solid state and in solution[14,15].

The only available infrared data are reported[16] without reference to their source or to the matrix in which they were recorded. The splitting of the CN stretching frequency in the i.r. spectrum might indicate that the symmetry is not perfectly octahedral. This lowering of the symmetry might be due to the presence of bulky ligands, as aromatic isocyanides are.

Although the reaction of $Re_2(CO)_{10}$ with isocyanides is not reported, chloropentacarbonylrhenium was treated with methyl and p-tolyl isocyanide[17]. While the reaction with the former was slow and incomplete, no reaction product being reported, the latter at 100° and in petroleum ether gave a stable, colourless, crystalline compound, formulated as $[Re(CO)_4(CNC_7H_7)_2]Cl$. This compound shows temperature-independent diamagnetism; its electrical conductivity in acetone is rather low for a strong uni–univalent electrolyte, though it is similar to that reported[17] for the related $[Re(CO)_4\text{-}py_2]Cl$. The isonitrile complex was found to be soluble in organic solvents; pyridine was effective in displacing the isocyanide at room temperature.

As with chloropentacarbonylmanganese derivatives, it is possible to have tetrasubstituted derivatives, but complete expulsion of carbon monoxide has not been reported, possibly because no solvent-assisted substitution reaction was tried. A refluxing benzene solution of p-tolyl isocyanide and $(CO)_2(PPh_3)_2ReX$ (X = Cl, Br) gave yellow $ReX(CO)(PPh_3)_2(CNC_7H_7)$, while heating at 180° afforded $ReCl(CO)(PPh_3)_2(C_7H_7NC)_2$, all diamagnetic non-electrolytes[18].

Rhenium (II) derivatives[19] were reported and characterized (see Table 5.2). On account of some recent additional physical evidence, previously not available, a reinvestigation is being carried out (M. Freni, personal communication).

Table 5.1 Isocyanide compounds of manganese

Name	Formula	Colour	M.p. °C	Uncorrected magnetic moment & other data[a]	Ref.
a) Derivatives of Mn(II)					
Hexakis(ethyl isocyanide) manganese (II) hexafluorophosphate	$[Mn(CNC_2H_5)_6](PF_6)_2$	Pink crystals	—	i.r.:2208	2
Hexakis(*t*-butyl isocyanide)-manganese (II) hexafluorophosphate	$[Mn(CNC_4H_9)_6](PF_6)_2$	White crystals	—	i.r.:2172	2
Hexakis(vinyl isocyanide)-manganese (II) tetrabromocadmiate	$[Mn(CNC_2H_3)_6]CdBr_4$	Dark red crystals	109	i.r.:2090	2
Hexakis(phenyl isocyanide)-manganese (II) tetrabromocadmiate	$[Mn(CNC_6H_5)_6]CdBr_4$	Violet crystals	—	i.r.:2090	2
Hexakis(*p*-tolylisocyanide)-manganese (II) nitrate	$[Mn(CNC_7H_7)_6](NO_3)_2$	Blue crystals	114	1·69	1
Hexakis(*p*-tolyl isocyanide)-manganese (II) perchlorate	$[Mn(CNC_7H_7)_6](ClO_4)_2$	Blue crystals	125	1·72	1
Hexakis(*p*-tolyl isocyanide)-manganese (II) tetrabromocadmiate	$[Mn(CNC_7H_7)_6][CdBr_4]$	Blue crystals	145	1·75 i.r.:2161 (nujol)	1, 3
Hexakis(*p*-anisyl isocyanide)-manganese (II) tetraiodomercurate	$[Mn(CNC_7H_7O)_6][HgI_4]$	Blue crystals	132	1·72	1
Hexakis(*p*-anisyl isocyanide)-manganese (II) picrate	$[Mn(CNC_7H_7O)_6][OC_6H_3(NO_2)_3]_2$	Blue crystals	116	1·74	1
b) Derivatives of Mn(I) with isonitriles as only ligands					
Hexakis(methyl isocyanide)-manganese (I) iodide	$[Mn(CNCH_3)_6]I$	White needles	263–264	[b]	3, 6
Hexakis(methyl isocyanide)-manganese (I) triiodide	$[Mn(CNCH_3)_6]I_3$	Light blue crystals	151–152	—	20
Hexakis(methyl isocyanide)-manganese (I) perchlorate	$[Mn(CNCH_3)_6]ClO_4$	White crystals	161 (dec.)	—	20
Hexakis(methyl isocyanide)-manganese (I) tetraphenylborate	$[Mn(CNCH_3)_6]B(C_6H_5)_4$	White needles	250–251	—	20
Hexakis(ethyl isocyanide)-manganese (I) iodide	$[Mn(CNC_2H_5)_6]I$	White needles	188–190	—	20

[a] If the matrix of the i.r. measurement is not given, it was absent in the original paper.
[b] ν(CN):2114 ± 15 (nujol), 2139 (CH_2Cl_2).

Table 5.1 (*continued*)

Name	Formula	Colour	M.p. °C	Uncorrected magnetic moment & other data[a]	Ref.
Hexakis(ethyl isocyanide)-manganese(I) triiodide	[Mn(CNC$_2$H$_5$)$_6$]I$_3$	Brown needles	272	—	20
Hexakis(ethyl isocyanide)-manganese(I) tetraphenylborate	[Mn(CNC$_2$H$_5$)$_6$][B(C$_6$H$_5$)$_4$]	White needles	134–135	—	20
Hexakis(ethyl isocyanide)-manganese(I) nitrate	[Mn(C$_2$H$_5$NC)$_6$]NO$_3$	White crystals		i.r.:2093	2
Hexakis(i-butyl isocyanide)-manganese(I) nitrate	[Mn(CNC$_4$H$_9$)$_6$]NO$_3$	White crystals	227–229	i.r.:2090, 2060	2
Hexakis(vinyl isocyanide)-manganese(I) nitrate	[Mn(CNC$_2$H$_3$)$_6$]NO$_3$	Yellow crystals	210	i.r.:2085	2
Hexakis(vinyl isocyanide)-manganese(I) iodide	[Mn(CNC$_2$H$_3$)$_6$]I	Yellow crystals	213·5–214·5	i.r.:2085	2
Hexakis(cyclohexyl isocyanide)-manganese(I) iodide	[Mn(CNC$_6$H$_{11}$)$_6$]I	White needles	140–142	—	20
Hexakis(cyclohexyl isocyanide)-manganese(I) triiodide	[Mn(CNC$_6$H$_{11}$)$_6$]I$_3$	Colourless crystals	68–69	—	20
Hexakis(cyclohexyl isocyanide)-manganese(I) tetraphenylborate	[Mn(CNC$_6$H$_{11}$)$_6$][B(C$_6$H$_5$)$_4$]	White needles	118–120	—	20
Hexakis(benzyl isocyanide)-manganese(I) iodide	[Mn(CNC$_7$H$_7$)$_6$]I	White crystals	184	—	20
Hexakis(benzyl isocyanide)-manganese(I) triiodide	[Mn(CNC$_7$H$_7$)$_6$]I$_3$	Red–brown crystals	115–116	—	20
Hexakis(benzyl isocyanide)-manganese(I) perchlorate	[Mn(CNC$_7$H$_7$)$_6$]ClO$_4$	White crystals	185–186	—	20
Hexakis(benzyl isocyanide)-manganese(I) tetraphenylborate	[Mn(CNC$_7$H$_7$)$_6$][B(C$_6$H$_5$)$_4$]	White crystals	128	—	20
Hexakis(phenyl isocyanide)-manganese(I) chloride	[Mn(CNC$_6$H$_5$)$_6$]Cl	Pale yellow	178	c	11
Hexakis(phenyl isocyanide)-manganese(I) iodide	[Mn(CNC$_6$H$_5$)$_6$]I	Yellow crystals	216	—	4
Hexakis(phenyl isocyanide)-(manganese(I) triiodide	[Mn(CNC$_6$H$_5$)$_6$]I$_3$	Brown crystals	164 (dec.)	—	4
Hexakis(phenyl isocyanide)-manganese(I) perchlorate	[Mn(CNC$_6$H$_5$)$_6$]ClO$_4$	Yellow crystals	213 (dec.)	—	4

Hexakis(phenyl isocyanide)manganese (I) nitrate	[Mn(CNC$_6$H$_5$)$_6$]NO$_3$	Yellow crystals		i.r.:2080	2
Hexakis(p-chlorophenyl isocyanide)manganese (I) iodide	[Mn(CNC$_6$H$_4$Cl)$_6$]I	Pale yellow crystals	247	—	4
Hexakis(p-chlorophenyl isocyanide)manganese (I) triiodide	[Mn(CNC$_6$H$_4$Cl)$_6$]I$_3$	Brown crystals	219 (dec.)	—	4
Hexakis(p-chlorophenyl isocyanide)manganese (I) perchlorate	[Mn(CNC$_6$H$_4$Cl)$_6$]ClO$_4$	Yellow crystals	235 (dec.)	—	4
Hexakis(p-tolyl isocyanide)manganese (I) iodide	[Mn(CNC$_7$H$_7$)$_6$]I	Pale yellow crystals	219	^{e} $-340 \times 10^{-6\,d}$ $29 \cdot 2^{\,f}$	4, 3
Hexakis(p-tolyl isocyanide)manganese (I) triiodide	[Mn(CNC$_7$H$_7$)$_6$]I$_3$	Brown crystals	184 (dec.)	$-790 \times 10^{-6\,d}$	4
Hexakis(p-tolyl isocyanide)manganese (I) perchlorate	[Mn(CNC$_7$H$_7$)$_6$]ClO$_4$	Pale yellow crystals	211 (dec.)	$-390 \times 10^{-6\,d}$ $30 \cdot 0^{\,f}$	4
Hexakis(p-anisyl cyanide)manganese (I) hydroxide	[Mn(CNC$_7$H$_7$O)$_6$]OH	Yellow crystals	—	—	6
Hexakis(p-anisyl isocyanide)manganese (I) chloride	[Mn(CNC$_7$H$_7$O)$_6$]Cl	Yellow crystals	182	—	4
Hexakis(p-anisyl isocyanide)manganese (I) bromide	[Mn(CNC$_7$H$_7$O)$_6$]Br	Yellow crystals	198	—	4
Hexakis(p-anisyl isocyanide)manganese (I) iodide	[Mn(CNC$_7$H$_7$O)$_6$]I	Pale yellow crystals	227	—	4
Hexakis(p-anisyl isocyanide)manganese (I) triiodide	[Mn(CNC$_7$H$_7$O)$_6$]I$_3$	Brown crystals	172	$-816 \times 10^{-6\,d}$	4
Hexakis(p-anisyl isocyanide)manganese (I) hydrogen carbonate	[Mn(CNC$_7$H$_7$O)$_6$]HCO$_3$	Pale yellow crystals	128 (dec.)	—	6
Hexakis(p-anisyl isocyanide)manganese (I) chlorate	[Mn(CNC$_7$H$_7$O)$_6$]ClO$_3$	Pale yellow crystals	118 (dec.)	—	6
Hexakis(p-anisyl isocyanide)manganese (I) perchlorate	[Mn(CNC$_7$H$_7$O)$_6$]ClO$_4$	Pale yellow crystals	213 (dec.)	$-440 \times 10^{-6\,d}$	4
Hexakis(p-anisyl isocyanide)manganese (I) tetrafluoroborate	[Mn(CNC$_7$H$_7$O)$_6$]BF$_4$	Pale yellow crystals	221	—	6

^{c} ν(CN); 2214vs, 2016s (KCl).

^{d} Magnetic susceptibility of the solid at 20° (χ_M).

^{e} ν(CN) in CHCl$_3$;2090, 2035w.

^{f} Molar conductivity, Λ_M in 1/5000 molar nitrobenzene solution at 18°.

Table 5.1 (*continued*)

Name	Formula	Colour	M.p. °C	Uncorrected magnetic moment & other data[a]	Ref.
Hexakis(p-anisyl isocyanide)manganese (I) tetraphenylborate	[Mn(CNC_7H_7O)_6]B(C_6H_5)_4	Pale yellow crystals	164	-710×10^{-6d} 19·1f	6
Hexakis(p-anisyl isocyanide)manganese (I) hexafluorophosphate	[Mn(CNC_7H_7O)_6]PF_6	Yellow crystals	207	—	6
c) Derivatives of Mn(I) with mixed ligands					
Chlorotricarbonyldi(p-anisyl isocyanide)manganese (I)	MnCl(CO)_3(CNC_7H_7O)_2	Ochre	—	—	12
π-Cyclopentadienyltri(phenyl isocyanide)manganese (I)	Mn(π-C_5H_5)(CNC_6H_5)_3	Yellow crystals	97	—	10
Bromotetracarbonyl(phenyl isocyanide)manganese (I)	MnBr(CO)_4(CNC_6H_5)	Yellow	pentane 86–87 methanol ligroin	2188w, 2107w, 2045s, 1993m, CCl_4	11
Bromotricarbonyldi(phenyl isocyanide)manganese (I)	MnBr(CO)_3(CNC_6H_5)_2	Pale yellow	84–86 pentane	2198m, 2174s, 2053s, 2004s, 1954s, KCl	11
Bromodicarbonyltri(phenyl isocyanide)manganese (I)	MnBr(CO)_2(CNC_6H_5)_3	Yellow	129–130 ether	2179w, 2214s, 2049s, 2020s, 1942s, KCl	11
Iodocarbonyltetrakis(phenyl isocyanide)manganese (I)	MnI(CO)(CNC_6H_5)_4	Yellow	171 ether	2088s, 1992m, 1894s, KCl	11
Bromocarbonyltetrakis(phenyl isocyanide)manganese (I)	MnBr(CO)(CNC_6H_5)_4	Orange	180 d. THF	2101vs, 2012m, 1919s, CCl_4	11
Bromopentakis(phenyl isocyanide)manganese (I)	MnBr(CNC_6H_5)_5	Colourless	213 d. THF	2101vs, 2012m, C_2H_4Cl_2	11
π-Cyclopentadienyldicarbonyl(phenyl isocyanide)manganese (I)	Mn(C_5H_5)(CO)_2(CNC_6H_{11})	Yellow	68–69	1949, 1898; $\mu(20°\text{C}_6\text{H}_6)$ 4·64 Debye	8, 9
cis-Bromotetracarbonyl(ethyl isocyanide)manganese (I)	MnCl(CO)_4(CNC_2H_5)	—	—	—	13
d) Manganese (o) derivatives					
Enneacarbonyl(phenyl isocyanide)dimanganese (o)	Mn_2(CO)_9(CNC_6H_5)	yellow	54 pentane	2169s, 2102s, 2045s, 2016s, 1980s, CCl_4	11
Octacarbonyldi(phenyl isocyanide)dimanganese (o)	Mn_2(CO)_8(CNC_6H_5)_2	yellow	111 pentane	2165vs, 2128m, 2061m, 2020m, 1966s, 1957m, CCl_4	11

Table 5.2 Isocyanide compounds of rhenium

Name	Formula	Colour and crystal form	M.p. °C	Other data[a]	Ref.
Rhenium (II) *derivatives*					
Iodobis(p-tolyl isocyanide)bis(triphenylphosphine)rhenium iodide	[ReI(C$_7$H$_7$NC)(C$_{18}$H$_{15}$P)$_2$]$_2$I	Orange	130	diamagn. $\Lambda = 19 \cdot 9$	18
The same, perchlorate	[ReI(C$_7$H$_7$NC)(C$_{18}$H$_{15}$P)$_2$]ClO$_4$	Pale brown	142	$\Lambda = 19 \cdot 5$	18
The same, periodide	[ReI(C$_7$H$_7$NC)(C$_{18}$H$_{15}$P)$_2$]I$_3$	Brown	140	$\Lambda = 14 \cdot 3$	18
The same, iodide	[ReI(C$_7$H$_7$NC)(C$_{18}$H$_{15}$P)$_2$]I	Yellow	232 dec.	$\Lambda = 27$ at 30°C	18
The same, tetraphenylborate	[ReI(C$_7$H$_7$NC)(C$_{18}$H$_{15}$P)$_2$][C$_{24}$H$_{20}$B]	Pale yellow	140	$\Lambda = 14 \cdot 7$	18
Rhenium (I) *derivatives*					
Chlorocarbonyl(p-tolyl isocyanide)bis(triphenylphosphine)rhenium	ReCl(CO)(C$_7$H$_7$NC)(C$_{18}$H$_{15}$P)$_2$	Yellow	200 dec.	diamagn. non-electr.	19
Bromocarbonyl[p-tolyl isocyanide)bis(triphenylphosphine)rhenium	ReBr(CO)(C$_7$H$_7$NC)(C$_{18}$H$_{15}$P)$_2$	Canary yellow	193	diamagn. non-electr.	19
Tetracarbonylbis(p-tolyl isocyanide)rhenium chloride	[Re(CO)$_4$(C$_7$H$_7$NC)$_2$]Cl	Colourless	>280 dec.	b,c	17
Carbonylbis(p-tolyl isocyanide)bis(triphenylphosphine)rhenium chloride	ReCl(CO)(C$_7$H$_7$NC)$_2$(PPh$_3$)$_2$	Canary yellow	200	—	19
Hexakis(ethyl isocyanide)rhenium periodide	[Re(C$_2$H$_5$NC)$_6$]I$_3$	Yellow brown	206	$\Lambda = 31$; $\chi = -380 \times 10^{-6}$	15
Hexakis(p-tolyl isocyanide)rhenium periodide	[Re(C$_7$H$_7$NC)$_6$]I$_3$	Yellow brown	170	$\Lambda = 18$; $\chi = -560 \times 10^{-6}$	15
The same, iodide	[Re(C$_7$H$_7$NC)$_6$]I	Yellow	238	$\Lambda = 27$; $\chi = -430 \times 10^{-6}$	15
The same, nitrate	[Re(C$_7$H$_7$NC)$_6$]NO$_3$	Yellow	206	$\Lambda = 27$; $\chi = -400 \times 10^{-6}$	15
The same, perchlorate	[Re(C$_7$H$_7$NC)$_6$]ClO$_4$	Yellow	241	$\Lambda = 27$; $\chi = -460 \times 10^{-6}$	15
The same, tetraphenylborate	[Re(C$_7$H$_7$NC)$_6$][C$_{24}$H$_{20}$B]	Pale yellow	215	$\Lambda = 23$; $\chi = -640 \times 10^{-6}$	15
The same, pentachlorotriphenylphosphinerhenate (IV)	[Re(C$_7$H$_7$NC)$_6$][ReCl$_5$(C$_{18}$H$_{15}$P)]	Orange–red	224	—	21
Rhenium (III) *derivatives*					
Trichloro(p-tolyl isocyanide)rhenium, dimer	[ReCl$_3$(C$_7$H$_7$NC)]$_2$	Dark red	79	diamagn. non-elec.	18
Triiodo(p-tolyl isocyanide)rhenium	ReI$_3$(C$_7$H$_7$NC)	Black	147	diamagn. non-elec.	18

[a] Λ is the electrical conductance of a 10^{-3} molar nitrobenzene solution at 16 or 20°C; χ is the magnetic susceptibility at 22°C (cc/mole).
[b] $\Lambda = 0 \cdot 50$ ohm^{-1} cm^{-2} mole, acetone, 832 liter/mole.
[c] Diamagnetic at 295 (-182×10^{-6}) and 195°K.

REFERENCES

1. L. Naldini, *Gazz. Chim. Ital.*, **90**, 871 (1960).
2. D. S. Matteson, personal communication (June 29, 1967).
3. F. A. Cotton and F. Zingales, *J. Am. Chem. Soc.*, **83**, 351 (1961).
4. A. Sacco, *Gazz. Chim. Ital.*, **86**, 201 (1956).
5. G. Winkhaus and H. Uhrig, *Z. analyt. Chem.*, **200**, 14 (1964).
6. A. Sacco and L. Naldini, *Gazz. Chim. Ital.*, **86**, 207 (1956).
7. A. Sacco and L. Naldini, *Ist. Lombardo (Rend. Sc.), Part I*, **91**, 288 (1957).
8. E. O. Fischer and M. Gerberhold, *Experientia*, Suppl., **9**, 259 (1964).
9. W. Strohmeier, J. F. Guttenberger and H. Hellmann, *Z. Naturforsch.*, **19b**, 353 (1964).
10. P. L. Pauson and W. H. Stubbs, *Angew. Chem.*, **74**, 466 (1962); *Angew. Chem. (Int. Edit.)*, **1**, 333 (1962).
11. K. K. Joshi, P. L. Pauson and W. H. Stubbs, *J. Organomet. Chem.*, **1**, 51 (1963).
12. W. Hieber and W. Scropp, Jr., *Z. Naturforsch.*, **14b**, 460 (1959).
13. R. J. Angelici and F. Basolo, *J. Am. Chem. Soc.*, **84**, 2495 (1962).
14. L. Malatesta, M. Freni, V. Valenti and E. Bossi, *Angew. Chem.*, **72**, 323 (1960).
15. M. Freni and V. Valenti, *Gazz. Chim. Ital.*, **91**, 1352 (1961).
16. R. D. Peacock, *The Chemistry of Technetium and Rhenium*, Elsevier, Amsterdam, 1966, p. 97.
17. W. Hieber and L. Schuster, *Z. anorg. Chem.*, **287**, 214 (1956).
18. M. Freni and V. Valenti, *Gazz. Chim. Ital.*, **90**, 1445 (1960).
19. M. Freni and V. Valenti, *Gazz. Chim. Ital.*, **90**, 1436 (1960).
20. A. Sacco, *Ann. Chim. (Italy)*, **48**, 225 (1958).
21. M. Freni, V. Valenti and R. Pomponi, *Gazz. Chim. Ital.*, **94**, 521 (1964).

6 ISOCYANIDE COMPLEXES OF IRON AND RUTHENIUM

IRON

Compounds obtained by alkylation of hexacyanoferrates

Though they are undoubtedly coordination compounds of isocyanides, some of them are formally considered as esters of hexacyanoferric (II) acid ('alkylferrocyanides'). The salts of the cation $[Fe(CNR)_6]^{2+}$ (R = methyl, ethyl, n-propyl) are the most important compounds of this class. The so-called 'alkylferrocyanides', of general formula $Fe(CN)_2(CNR)_4$, are interesting because they occur in isomeric forms, the several structures of which have not yet been fully established. Owing to the complexity of the matter, a somewhat chronological order will be adopted in the description of these compounds.

In the last decades of the nineteenth century, a great deal of interest was shown by organic chemists in the structure of potassium hexacyanoferrate (II) (potassium ferrocyanide) to which, among others, the following structures were attributed[1]:

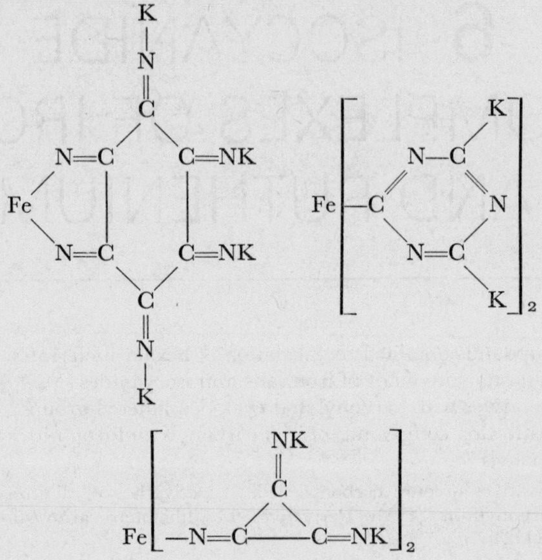

$$
\begin{array}{c}
K \\
| \\
N \\
\| \\
C \\
\end{array}
$$

Fe

$$
\begin{array}{cc}
N=C & C=NK \\
N=C & C=NK
\end{array}
$$

$$
\begin{array}{c}
C \\
\| \\
N \\
| \\
K
\end{array}
$$

$$
Fe \left[\begin{array}{cc} N-C & \\ C & N \\ N=C & \\ & K \end{array} \right]_2
$$

$$
Fe \left[-N=C \overset{\overset{NK}{\underset{\|}{C}}}{\diagdown} C=NK \right]_2
$$

In order to determine its structure, many attempts were made to obtain organic derivatives of potassium hexacyanoferrate (II). The esterification of the corresponding free acid was attempted in 1854 by Buff[2] who, by treating hexacyanoferric (II) acid with hydrogen chloride in alcohol, obtained a product which was formulated as $(C_2H_5)_4Fe(CN)_6 . 2 C_2H_5Cl . 6 H_2O$. This product was later shown[3,4] to have the character of an iminoether, so that it could be written as

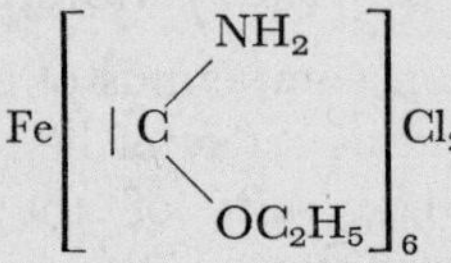

$$
Fe \left[| \; C \overset{\diagup NH_2}{\underset{\diagdown OC_2H_5}{}} \right]_6 Cl_2 \quad \text{or} \quad 4EtOH.H_4Fe(CN)_6 + 2EtOH.HCl4
$$

However, the method is capable of giving the desired product and indeed Heldt[5] has obtained an isonitrile complex by heating hexacyanoferric (II) acid with an alcohol in an autoclave.

The first true isocyanoiron derivative isolated in a pure state was Freund's 'ethylferrocyanide' (1888) which was prepared by treating silver hexacyanoferrate (II) with ethyl iodide[4]. At that time it was written as $(C_2H_5)_4Fe(CN)_6$, but as it gives off isocyanide on addition of potassium cyanide or on heating, and shows no electrical conductance in solution, it must be considered to be dicyanotetrakis-(ethyl isocyanide)iron (II), $Fe(CN)_2(CNC_2H_5)_4$.

The methylation reaction of ferrocyanides was extensively studied by Hartley. The results of his research, described in a long series of papers (1910–1933), is summarized in the pages which follow. It must be stressed that here we attribute to Hartley's compounds the structure of isocyanide coordination compounds, which he took into consideration only in 1933.

The 'esterification reaction' is carried out by refluxing for several hours a mixture of dry and finely powdered potassium hexa-cyanoferrate (II) with freshly distilled dimethyl sulphate[6]. The reaction mixture is then filtered hot; on cooling the solution, a pre-cipitate separates, which, after recrystallization from methanol, has a composition corresponding to the formula $[Fe(CNCH_3)_6](HSO_4)_2$ (1).

This product is slightly soluble in alcohol and gives a precipitate with barium salts. From the mother liquor of 1, after removing the excess of dimethyl sulphate by evaporating it under reduced pressure, a crystalline mass is obtained. After recrystallization from methanol, it analyses as $[Fe(CNCH_3)_6]$ $(CH_3SO_4)_2 . 2$ CH_3HSO_4 (2). This product is readily soluble in alcohol and gives no precipitate with barium salts. In vacuum it changes slowly into 1:

$$[Fe(CNCH_3)_6](CH_3SO_4)_2(CH_3HSO_4)_2 \rightarrow$$
$$[Fe(CNCH_3)_6](HSO_4)_2 + 2 (CH_3)_2SO_4$$

When the methylation reaction was carried out under different conditions, another compound was obtained—$[Fe(CNCH_3)_6]$-$(CH_3SO_4)_2$ (3). The compounds 1, 2 and 3 give the same precipitate, $[Fe(CNCH_3)_6][PtCl_6]$, with hexachloroplatinic (IV) acid, which proves that they are salts of the same cation, $[Fe(CNCH_3)_6]^{2+}$.

The methylation reaction described above can be formally written as follows

$$[Fe(CN)_6]^{4-} + 6 (CH_3)^+ \rightarrow [Fe(CNCH_3)_6]^{2+}$$

thus stressing the intimate relations between cyanometallates and isocyanide coordination compounds.

The salt 1 is the most easily obtained because of its sparing solu-bility, and is also formed by treating alcoholic solutions of 2 and 3 with sulphuric acid.

By neutralizing a solution of 1 with barium hydroxide the sulphate 4 is formed. This can be isolated but, being very soluble, cannot easily be obtained in a pure state. From the sulphate **4** the chloride **5** can be prepared as follows. A solution of the sulphate is treated with a slight excess of barium chloride, filtered and evaporated to dryness under reduced pressure. The residue is extracted with alcohol and the alcoholic solution precipitated with ether. The chloride separates in a bulky colourless crystalline mass:

$$[Fe(CNCH_3)_6](HSO_4)_2 + Ba(OH)_2 \rightarrow [Fe(CNCH_3)_6]SO_4 + BaSO_4 + 2\,H_2O$$
$$\text{(1)} \qquad\qquad\qquad\qquad\qquad \text{(4)}$$

$$[Fe(CNCH_3)_6]SO_4 + BaCl_2 \rightarrow [Fe(CNCH_3)_6]Cl_2 + BaSO_4$$
$$\text{(5)}$$

According to Hoelzl (1927)[7], the chloride **5** can also be prepared by boiling an aqueous solution of **1**, **2** or **3** with HCl or $BaCl_2$. No ion-exchange resin was available in those days.

Controlled alkylation of dicyanotetrakis(methyl isocyanide)iron with methyl iodide gave cyanopentakis(methyl isocyanide)iron (II) iodide, together with some hexakis(methyl isocyanide)iron (II) iodide[8].

Hexakis(methyl isocyano)iron (II) chloride was the first isocyanide derivative of which the structure was fully determined. Powell and Bartindale[9] found in 1945 a value of 1·85 Å for the carbon–iron distance, rather lower than the value calculated from the covalent radii of the elements and very near to that in $Fe(CO)_5$. From this value, the amount of double bonding in the carbon–iron link was estimated to be about 50%. It was also shown that the bonds Fe—C—N—CH_3 are not on a straight line, but there might be a bend with a C—N—C angle of 7 degrees. However, the accuracy of this study is rather low (see p. 29) by present standards.

When it is heated under reduced pressure at 130–150°, the chloride of hexakis(methyl isocyanide)iron (II) is transformed into the 'methylferrocyanide', that is, into the dicyanotetrakis(methyl isocyanide)iron (II) (**6**), which is the methyl analogue of Freund's 'ethylferrocyanide':

$$[Fe(CNCH_3)_6]Cl_2 \xrightarrow{150°} Fe(CN)_2(CNCH_3)_4 + 2\,CH_3Cl$$

This compound cannot be prepared directly from $Ag_4[Fe(CN)_6]$ and CH_3I because, even with a defect of CH_3I, an addition compound between silver iodide and the iodide of hexakis(methyl isocyanide)iron (II) is obtained[10]:

$$Ag_4[Fe(CN)_6] + 6\,CH_3I \rightarrow [Fe(CNCH_3)_6]I_2 \cdot 4\,AgI$$

This double salt is decomposed by dilute nitric acid and silver nitrate:

$$[Fe(CNCH_3)_6]I_2 \cdot 4\,AgI \xrightarrow{\frac{HNO_3}{AgNO_3}} [Fe(CNCH_3)_6](NO_3)_2 + 6\,AgI$$

An analogous addition compound is formed in the reaction between silver hexacyanoferrate (II) and ethyl iodide[11], carried out at ordinary temperature. The adduct $[Fe(CNC_2H_5)_6]I_2 \cdot 4\,AgI$ gives with silver nitrate the salt $[Fe(CNC_2H_5)_6](NO_3)_2$ and with sulphuric acid the bisulphate, $[Fe(CNC_2H_5)_6](HSO_4)_2$.

In the reaction between silver hexacyanoferrate (III) (ferricyanide) and methyl iodide[10] some hexakis(methyl isocyanide)iron (II) triiodide is formed, together with the addition product with silver iodide:

$$4\,Ag_3[Fe(CN)_6] + 24\,CH_3I \rightarrow 3\,[Fe(CNCH_3)_6]I_2 \cdot 4\,AgI + [Fe(CNCH_3)_6](I_3)_2$$

A better preparation of another halide was reported by Malhotra[8] who alkylated $K_4[Fe(CN)_6]$ with excess methyl bromide.

The dicyanotetrakis(methyl isocyanide)iron (II), mentioned above, is not a single product, but a mixture of two isomers, called α and β, which can be separated owing to their different solubilities in chloroform[12]. By alkylation with methyl iodide, the two isomers give the same cation, $[Fe(CNCH_3)_6]^{2+}$; when ethyl iodide instead of methyl iodide is used, two different cations are obtained[11]. These facts, together with the known molecular weights in solution, agree with the suggestion[13] that the α and β-forms of the 'tetramethyl-ferrocyanide' are *cis* and *trans* isomers, and Powell and Stanger showed by x-ray examination that the β-form is the *trans* hexaco-ordinated compound[14].

It may be interesting to recall that during these x-ray investigations on isocyanide compounds Powell observed that the isocyanide–iron bonds were strictly similar to those of the mononuclear carbonyls. Considering that one of the reasons for the stability of compounds of this type is the attainment of the effective atomic number of the next noble gas, he foresaw that compounds such as $Mn(CN)$-$(CNCH_3)_5$ and $Cr(CNCH_3)_6$ should be capable of existence. In fact, isocyanide compounds very similar to those predicted by Powell were obtained later.

In addition to the 'α- and β-tetramethylferrocyanides' of Hartley, already mentioned[12], other supposed isomers and similar compounds have been described, but in our opinion their identification and formulation are rather uncertain. Hoelzl repeated[7] the preparation of the 'methylferrocyanides' in a way slightly different from Hartley's and obtained two substances, which he called α and β and considered to be the same as Hartley's α- and β-isomers. For the former he objected to the structure of dicyanotetrakis(methyl isocyanide)iron (II) and formulated it as a dicyanide of tetrakis(methyl isocyanide)-iron (II). However, Hoelzl's β-isomer was later recognized[11] to be different from Hartley's, for which a structure trans-dicyanotetrakis-(methyl isocyanide)iron (II) was found by x-ray investigation[14]. Hoelzl's β-isomer, according to a proposal of Meyer[15], has since been called γ. The 'γ-methylferrocyanide' is a substance that is more soluble in water than the β-form, is nearly insoluble in chloroform and behaves as an electrolyte.

There are two other substances with a composition similar to the α, β and γ-isomers. One was obtained by Meyer and coworkers[15] by treating hexacyanoferric (II) acid with diazomethane. It was a salt-like product which analysed as $(CH_3)_4Fe(CN)_6 . H_2O$ and was formulated as a cyanide of cyanoaquotetrakis(methyl isocyanide)iron (II), $[Fe(CN)(H_2O)(CNCH_3)_4]CN$. The other was obtained by Hoelzl[7], by extracting the solid mass obtained in the preparation of $[Fe(CNCH_3)_6]Cl_2$ with aqueous instead of anhydrous methanol. The aqueous alcoholic solution was evaporated under reduced pressure and the residue heated under vacuum at 150–160°; the substance thus obtained was an electrolyte of composition corresponding to $Fe(CN)_2(CNCH_3)_4 . 4 H_2O . 2 CH_3OH$. It was formulated by Hoelzl as a dicyanide of bis(methanolo)tetrakis(methyl isocyanide)iron (II) tetrahydrate, $[Fe(CH_3OH)_2(CNCH_3)_4](CN)_2 . 4 H_2O$, but it seems very strange, to say the least, that a compound obtained by heating under vacuum should contain methanol and water.

From the reaction between silver hexacyanoferrate (II) and n-propyl iodide, Hoelzl could isolate[7] only one of the possible isomers of the dicyanotetrakis(n-propyl isocyanide)iron (II):

$$Ag_4[Fe(CN)_6] + 4 C_3H_7I \rightarrow Fe(CN)_2(CNC_3H_7)_4 + 4 AgI$$

The product obtained is a white crystalline substance, soluble in alcohol and chloroform.

Hoelzl also described some hydrolysis products of 'methylferro-cyanide'; the best defined of these is a red (?) dicyanoaquotris(methyl isocyanide)iron (II), $Fe(CN)_2(H_2O)(CNCH_3)_3$[7].

Finally Meyer and coworkers[15] obtained compounds in which only one cyanide group had been alkylated by treating an ethereal solution of hexacyanoferric (III) acid with diazomethane and diazoethane. The free acids $H_2[Fe(CN)_5(CNCH_3)]$ and $H_2[Fe(CN)_5(CNC_2H_5)]$ are very unstable, but their silver and copper salts, and in general the salts with cations of heavy metals, though not easily obtained in a pure state, seem to be quite stable.

Recently much work in this field has been published by Heldt both in journals and in patents[16,17]; a review by the same author[18] is available. A convenient method was described for the preparation of very stable pentakis(isocyanide)cyanoiron halides and of many other salts from alkali ferrocyanides and alkyl halides, activated in the α-position (e.g. alkyl, benzyl). The probable reaction mechanism[19] is the displacement of the halide from the alkyl halide by the ferro-cyanide anion or the partially alkylated ferrocyanide anion. Both the ionization of the alkyl halide and the nucleophilicity of the anion appear to influence the rate of the reaction.

The reaction of pentakis(benzyl isocyanide)cyanoiron bromide with various nucleophiles was studied in detail[20]. Strong nucleo-philic agents, such as sodium hydroxide or sodium bicarbonate, give only tarry polymers. Potassium cyanide causes polymer formation and liberates benzyl isocyanide. Weak bases which form only moderately stable complexes with iron (II), such as methanol, ammonia or ethyl mercaptan, were benzylated. Taking advantage of the readily available $[(C_6H_5CH_2NC)_5FeCN]^+$ or $(C_6H_5CH_2NC)_4Fe(CN)_2$, their reaction with an alkyl halide was studied, with continuous removal of the benzyl halide formed. By a reaction similar to the transesterification reaction a series of products with general formulae $[(R'NC)_x(C_6H_5CH_2NC)_yFeCN]X$ ($x + y$ = 5; X = halogen), $[(R'NC)_5FeBr]Br$ and $(R'NC)_4Fe(CN)_2$ was formed. Directions for the isolation of the individual products from the complex reaction mixture are given in detail[21]. The compounds even include derivatives of phenacyl isocyanide.

Some organic reactions of coordinated isocyanide were also studied by Heldt. Nitration, sulphonation, alkylation and bromina-tion of the very stable pentakis(benzyl isocyanide)cyanoiron hy-drogensulphate and tetrakis(benzyl isocyanide)dicyanoiron almost exclusively yielded products in which the electrophilic group entered the *para* position; the rate of the nitration was found to be 350 times faster than the nitration of benzene. An anchimeric assistance by the nitrogen in the transition state of aromatic electrophilic substitutions was invoked, since the main resonance structure of the isocyanide group complexed to iron (II) appears to be

$$C_5H_5CH_2N^\oplus ::: C:Fe^\ominus$$

and hence the aromatic groups should be strongly deactivated in this type of aromatic substitution. Additional support to this view was found by Heldt in the observation that addition of a strong Lewis acid, such as $AlCl_3$, makes the anchimeric assistance ineffective by complexing with the lone electron-pair on the nitrogen[22].

Other organic reactions studied on the same complexes included the condensation with aliphatic aldehydes in 96% sulphuric acid. The expected substituted benzyl alcohols were formed at first; then, by elimination of water, oligo- and polymeric materials were formed[23].

Few physical data are available on the $[(RNC)_6Fe]^{2+}$ and related derivatives. However, in recent times, Heldt collected infrared data reported in Table 6.1 and some n.m.r. data[24]; the electrical conductivity of the solid compounds was also investigated[25].

The polarographic data reported by Heldt on the reduction of $L_4Fe(CN)_2$, $[L_5Fe(CN)]HSO_4$ and $[L_6Fe]SO_4$ (L = benzyl isocyanide) did not allow any definite conclusion to be reached[24]. Other authors[26] found, during the polarographic reduction of hexakis(methyl isocyanide)iron dichloride in aqueous KCl, two polarographic waves. The first one (-1.52 volt, against s.c.e.) was assigned to direct reduction of Fe^{II} to metallic iron; the second was assigned either to the reduction of RNC to secondary amine or to hydrogen discharge. The same group of workers recorded the i.r. spectra of the complex, both in the hydrated and in the anhydrous ($+150°C$) state[27].

Another recent study, by Carassiti[28], gives data on the thermal and photochemical decomposition of hexakis(methyl isocyanide)iron (II) dichloride. Irradiation with light of fixed wavelength (254 and 365 mμ) of an aqueous solution brings about substitution of the isocyanide ligands with molecules of water, in a manner similar to that observed with hexacyanoferrate (II) salts[29]. Moreover, in both cases, irradiation of the solution of the complex with light having a wavelength corresponding to that of a La Porte forbidden, spin allowed d–d transition, produces the relatively stable $[FeL_4(H_2O)_2]^{2+}$ ion intermediately (L = CH_3NC). The quantum yields were 0.09 ($\lambda = 254$) and 0.03 ($\lambda = 365$).

Addition compounds of iron salts and isocyanides

The most interesting compounds of this class derive from iron (II) salts. They are all diamagnetic. The strong ligand field produced by the isonitrile ligands makes it possible for a singlet state arising from one of the free-ion states to drop far enough to become the ground state. These low-spin complexes are to be compared with $[Fe(CN)_6]^{4-}$ and $[Fe(phen)_3]^{24}$. The compounds obtained by direct reaction of iron (II) salts and isocyanides contain at most four molecules of ligand; no hexaisocyanide derivatives of the type described on p. 100 have been obtained so far. In these compounds, the coordination number of iron can be either four, as in $[Fe(CNR)_4](ClO_4)_2$, or six, as in $FeCl_2(CNR)_4$. Both the tetra- and hexacoordinated complexes are diamagnetic.

According to work of Hofmann and Bugge[30], it is possible to prepare addition compounds of $FeCl_3$ and isocyanides, though they are unstable and completely hydrolyzed by water. On the other hand, the analogous addition compounds of $FeCl_2$ are said to be quickly oxidized by air to derivatives of Fe (III).

The following compounds have been described: $FeCl_3 . 2 \ C_2H_5NC$ and $FeCl_3 . 3 \ C_2H_5NC$, yellow hygroscopic crystals, readily decomposed by alcohols, obtained by addition of isocyanides to an ethereal solution of $FeCl_3$; $Fe_2Cl_4O . 4 \ C_2H_5NC$ and $Fe_2Cl_4O . 5 \ C_2H_5NC$, unstable yellow crystalline substances, obtained from a methanolic or ethanolic solution of $FeCl_2$ and ethyl isocyanide (in the presence of air as oxidizing agent). They give both the reactions of Fe^{3+} and Cl^- free ions.

The real existence of these derivatives of iron (III) formed by spontaneous oxidation from iron (II) compounds should, however, be accepted with reserve. In fact, the reported tendency of the isocyanide derivatives to be oxidized by air is in contrast to the remarkable stability of both the hexakis(alkyl isocyanide)iron (II) salts of Hartley[1,6,31] and the tetraisocyanide compounds of Malatesta and coworkers[32].

By reacting anhydrous ferrous sulphate or ferrous chloride with alkyl and aryl isocyanides, without solvent or in ethereal suspension, Malatesta obtained[33] some addition compounds of composition corresponding to $FeSO_4 . 2 \ CNR$ and $FeCl_2 . 2 \ CNR$. These are yellow crystalline powders, extremely soluble in water, alcohol and polar organic solvents, by which they are readily decomposed. Their solutions give the reactions of SO_4^{2-} and Cl^- immediately, but not those of the Fe^{2+} ion. Their structures have not been investigated further.

When the reaction between iron (II) salts and isocyanides was carried out in alcoholic or aqueous alcoholic solution, very stable compounds of composition corresponding to $FeX_2(CNR)_4$ (X = Cl, Br, I, SCN; R = alkyl or aryl) were obtained (Malatesta and co-workers[32]). Similar compounds were also prepared from iron tetra-carbonyl dihalide and isocyanide[34].

All these compounds occur in two forms. One, obtained by rapid precipitation from cold solution, is intensely coloured (green or blue), and sparingly soluble; the other, obtained from the former by boiling it in the presence of solvents or directly by precipitation from hot solutions, is brown or yellow and very soluble in organic solvents. Both forms are diamagnetic and non-electrolytes, and, although their molecular weights have not been determined, they were assumed to be monomeric hexacoordinate *cis–trans* isomers, of the same type as the ' α- and β-methylferrocyanides' of Hartley. The point was confirmed later by recording the infrared spectra of some of these compounds in the CN stretching region[34,35]; in the case of benzyl isocyanide derivatives, raman and n.m.r. data are also available[24].

The aromatic analogues of 'methylferrocyanides' could not be prepared directly from $Fe(CN)_2$ and aryl isocyanides, probably because of the highly complex structure of the so-called ferrous cyanide. However, by reacting the dibromotetrakis(p-chlorophenyl isocyano)iron (II) with silver cyanide, two substances were obtained, one white and practically insoluble in chloroform, the other yellow and soluble in chloroform. Both had a composition corresponding to $Fe(CN)_2(CNC_6H_4Cl)_4$, and it is possible, though not proved, that they are the aromatic analogues of 'methylferrocyanides'. Here also, later infrared and n.m.r. evidence on the benzylisocyanide derivatives was in agreement with the hypothesis[24]. The high value of CN stretching frequency in these complexes is in agreement with the high oxidation number of the cation and with the absence of back-donation.

Sacco and Coletti[36], by reaction of ferrous halogenides with the potassium salts of p-isocyanobenzenesulphonic acid in alcoholic solution, obtained compounds of formula $K_4[FeX_2(CNC_6H_4SO_3)_4]$. These are crystalline substances, soluble in water but insoluble in organic solvents, by which they are slowly decomposed.

The dihalogenotetraisocyanoiron (II) compounds form stable and well-defined adducts with mercuric halides[32]. These compounds, of general formula $FeX_2(CNR)_4 \cdot HgX'_2$ (X and X' are the same or different halogen atoms) are red or brown-red crystalline substances, readily soluble in organic solvents. They can be considered similar to the addition compounds of hexakis(methyl isocyanide) iron (II) salts and silver or mercury (II) halides. No other data are available.

An interesting series of compounds was prepared by Padoa, by direct reaction of isocyanides and ferrous perchlorate, without solvents[37]. The reaction mixture, recrystallized several times from methanol, gave pale yellow crystals, of composition corresponding to $[Fe(CNR)_4](ClO_4)_2$ (R = phenyl, p-tolyl, p-chlorophenyl). These compounds are soluble in water, alcohol, chloroform and nitrobenzene, insoluble in benzene and ether. They have the character of strong uni-divalent electrolytes and are diamagnetic. They were attributed a tetracoordinated structure implying square planar dsp^2 hybrid orbitals.

Derivatives with carbonyl and cyclopentadienyl groups

Direct introduction of phenyl isocyanide in $C_5H_5Fe(CO)_2X$ was found possible[38,39]. When X = I the reaction was carried out in refluxing benzene; the main product was brown $C_5H_5Fe(CO)$-$(CNPh)I$ (35%), together with red $C_5H_5Fe(CNPh)_2I$ (8%), a trace of ferrocene and much unreacted starting material (53%). The same reaction on the bromide gave purple $C_5H_5Fe(CNPh)_2Br$ in 37% yield, while the chloride gave orange, ionic $[C_5H_5Fe(CNPh)_3]Cl$. This behaviour is similar to that towards reaction with triphenylphosphine: the iodide gives addition and substitution products, while the chloride gives mainly ionic substitution products.

When $C_5H_5Fe(CO)LI$ was reacted with PhNC in the same conditions, the starting material was recovered (89%) when L = CNPh, whereas a reaction was observed when L = PPh_3. Chromatographic separation of the reaction mixture afforded unreacted starting material (9%), a similar quantity of C_5H_5-$Fe(CO)(CNPh)I$ and $C_5H_5Fe(CNPh)_2I$ (42%)[38].

Another synthetic approach is available[40]. Reaction of the easily available $K[Fe(CN)_2(C_5H_5)(CO)]$ with a variety of alkyl bromides or iodides gave either of the two following reactions, according to the molar ratio of reagents:

$$K[Fe(CN)_2(C_5H_5)(CO)] + RX \rightarrow Fe(CN)(C_5H_5)(CO)(CNR) + KX$$

$$K[Fe(CN)_2(C_5H_5)(CO)] + 2\,RX \rightarrow [Fe(C_5H_5)(CO)(CNR)_2]X + KX$$

The reaction was carried out in refluxing acetonitrile. R included allyl, benzyl, p-chlorobenzyl and triphenylmethyl in the former case, only methyl, allyl and benzyl in the latter. The compounds are stable: the p-carbethoxybenzylisocyanide derivative was hydrolyzed (100°, 0·4 M HCl, 6 hr) to the corresponding acid in 52% yield.

A similar reaction might be possible with other organometallic iodides, yielding compounds analogous to those prepared by King[41] with Group VI elements. In consideration of this recent work, it is also possible that the reported yellow $H[Fe(CN)_2(C_5H_5)$-$CO]$[40] might be a neutral complex of HNC, instead of an acid. Infrared data were recorded for many of these compounds, and they are useful mainly for identification purposes.

When cyclopentadienylcarbonyl(phenyl isocyanide)iodoiron (II) was reduced[42] with an excess of $NaBH_4$ in refluxing tetrahydrofuran, chromatographic separation of the products gave ferrocene (16%), bis(cyclopentadienyldicarbonyliron) (8·4%) and the first isocyanide-bridged complex known, μ-carbonyl-μ-phenylisocyanide-bis-(cyclopentadienylcarbonyliron) (5·3%), together with a trace of a possible bis[carbonylcyclopentadienyl(phenyl isocyanide)iron]. The infrared spectrum of the isocyanide-bridged compound shows two bands (1704 and 1795 cm^{-1}) assigned to the bridging isocyanide and carbonyl groups; the value found for the CN stretching of bridging isocyanide is comparable with that of bis(carbonylcyclopentadienylnickel) (1785 cm^{-1}). The evidence for the structure includes an x-ray crystallographic examination (see Figure). No other evidence has yet become available about the structure in solutions. The related $[C_5H_5M(CO)_2]_2$ (M = Fe, Ru, Os) and

$C_5H_5Ni(CNR)_2$ give rise to interesting phenomena of equilibrium between bridged and non-bridged forms in solution.

Substitution compounds of iron carbonyls and iron nitrosylcarbonyls

Derivatives of pure carbonyls

Unlike nickel tetracarbonyl and dicobalt octacarbonyl, iron pentacarbonyl shows very low reactivity toward isocyanides. No reaction takes place in the cold when $Fe(CO)_5$ is treated with isocyanides, and the first attempts to carry out the reaction at higher temperature gave only 'sticky crusts that could not be recrystallized'[43]. The reaction between iron dodecacarbonyl and isocyanides, by contrast, proceeds rapidly and neatly[44]. The products are well-defined crystalline substances, corresponding to the substitution of one or two carbon monoxide molecules of $Fe(CO)_5$ by isocyanides:

$$[Fe(CO)_4]_3 + 3\,RNC \rightarrow 3\,Fe(CO)_4(CNR)$$

$$[Fe(CO)_4]_3 + 6\,RNC \rightarrow 3\,Fe(CO)_3(CNR_2) + 3\,CO$$

The same products can be obtained from iron pentacarbonyl at 70–90°, provided the isocyanide does not exceed the amount required by the above reactions. Even trimethyl(iso)cyanogermane, trimethyl(iso)cyanosilane and trimethyltin (iso)cyanide react, at this temperature[45], to yield yellow $LFe(CO)_4$. Low yields of $(PhNC)Fe(CO)_4$ were obtained by reaction of iron pentacarbonyl and PhNCS in refluxing cyclohexane[46].

Carbonylisocyanoiron compounds are yellow crystalline substances with low melting points. The monosubstituted compounds are remarkably volatile, though less so than the corresponding pure carbonyl, and are usually purified by sublimation in high vacuum. The disubstituted compounds are still volatile, but to a much lesser extent; both the mono- and the disubstituted compounds are photosensitive, moderately stable to air, soluble in organic solvents and insoluble in water. Their solutions have no electrical conductance, and the molecular weights in solution correspond to a monomeric structure.

The compounds with $(CH_3)_3MNC$ (M = Si, Ge, Sn) as ligands have similar properties; however, they are very air sensitive. They were considered isocyanide, and not cyanide, complexes, since the reaction of $Fe(CO)_5$ with nitriles gives different products, which are red and ionic, like $[Fe(N\equiv CC_6H_5)_n][Fe_3(CO)_n]$. Uncharacterized oily products of this type were indeed present, in the reaction mixture from which yellow $(CH_3)_3SnNCFe(CO)_4$ was isolated in low yields. Although it is not clear whether the red-brown and ionic oil is a product of the decomposition of the yellow complex or another primary reaction product, the difference between silicon- and germanium-containing iron derivatives on one hand, and tin-containing iron derivatives on the other, is in line with the difference between the properties of $(CH_3)_3M(CN)$ (M = Ge, Si) and of the polar $(CH_3)_3Sn(CN)$[47].

The intermediate formation of isocyanide complexes is essential in the metal–carbonyl–catalysed conversion of isocyanates to carbodiimides[48]:

$$Fe(CO)_5 + R—NCO \rightarrow Fe(CO)_4(CNR) + CO_2$$
$$Fe(CO)_4(CNR) + R—NCO \rightarrow RN{=}C{=}NR + Fe(CO)_5$$

The possibility of the first step was already known, since isocyanide complexes had been isolated by the reaction of metal carbonyls and phenyl isocyanate or isothiocyanate[46]. However, the conversion of the isocyanate to carbodiimide was high (80%). Many carbonyls (Fe, Mo, W) as well as $Fe(CO)_4(CNC_6H_5)$, were found effective catalysts and the quantity required was around 1% by weight.

Owing to the trigonal bipyramidal structure attributed to iron pentacarbonyl[49], the compounds of the type $Fe(CO)_3(CNR)_2$ were assumed to be able to exist in stereoisomeric forms. Hieber[50], however, obtained only one mixed disubstituted product, operating in the following two ways:

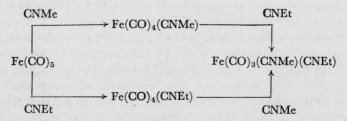

Since the bipyramidal structure is now proved for iron penta-carbonyl, the fact that no stereoisomers are obtained in the above reactions may be explained by assuming either that the two isocyanide molecules enter in equivalent positions or that they are easily interchanged.

The question was clarified later by Cotton[51,52]. He recorded the infrared spectra of $LFe(CO)_4$ and $L_2Fe(CO)_3$, where L included alkyl, phenyl, trimethylsilyl- and trimethylgermyl-isocyanide. From comparison with selection rules it was concluded that the configurations are very probably trigonal bipyramidal and that, when two L ligands are present, these lie on the two equivalent axial positions (that is, on the 3-fold axis of symmetry) of the molecule.

Examination of the values found for the CN stretching frequency in the $LFe(CO)_4$ compounds showed that there is practically no back-donation when L is a common aliphatic or aromatic isocyanide. The conclusion is in agreement with the value of the dipole moment, 5.07 or 5.02 D (if $P_A = 0.2 P_E$). The high value, to be compared with 3.5 D for isocyanides, suggests independently the virtual non-existence of back-donation and a polar bond, $\overset{\ominus}{M} \leftarrow C{\equiv}\overset{\oplus}{N}-R$, if the $CNCH_3$ moiety is linear[53].

However, for organosilicon or organogermanium isocyanide, back-donation dominates, as evidenced by the lowering of the CN-bond order. The difference was then interpreted as due to the presence on silicon and germanium of empty d orbitals and to the consequent stabilization of the entire group of π-electrons[51].

Derivatives of dinitrosyldicarbonyliron

Dinitrosyldicarbonyliron, $Fe(NO)_2(CO)_2$, which is isoelectronic with $Ni(CO)_4$, reacts with isocyanides much more readily than iron pentacarbonyl. The reaction consists in the displacement of the two CO molecules by two isocyanides, to give the dinitrosyldiisocyanide-iron compounds (method 1):

$$Fe(NO)_2(CO)_2 + 2\ RNC \rightarrow Fe(NO)_2(CNR)_2 + 2\ CO$$

The same products can also be obtained (2) from nitrosyl compounds of iron with isocyanides and (3) from the reaction of the dihalogeno-tetraisocyanide iron compounds with hydroxylamine.

The compounds containing methyl and ethyl isocyanide were prepared with the first method, carrying out the reaction in an inert atmosphere; the compounds containing aryl isocyanides can also be prepared by method 1, but were first obtained with methods 2 and 3[54,55].

The reactions with isocyanides of $K_2[Fe_2(NO)_4S_2]$, red Roussin's salt, and of $NH_4[Fe(NO)_2(S_2O_3)]$ are examples of method 2:

$$K_2[Fe_2(NO)_4S_2] + 4\ RNC \rightarrow 2\ Fe(NO)_2(CNR)_2 + K_2S_2$$

$$NH_4[Fe(NO)_2(S_2O_3)] + 2\ RNC \rightarrow Fe(NO)_2(CNR)_2 + \tfrac{1}{2}\ (NH_4)_2S_4O_6$$

The reaction takes place in alcohol upon gently warming the mixture. The products can be purified by dissolution in benzene followed by reprecipitation with alcohol.

Method 3 is based on the fact, pointed out by Nast[56], that hydroxylamine in alkaline solution undergoes a disproportionation reaction:

$$2 NH_2OH \rightarrow NH_3 + NOH + H_2O$$

$$NOH \rightarrow NO^- + H^+$$

$$FeX_2(CNR)_4 + 2 NO^- \rightarrow Fe(NO)_2(CNR)_2 + 2 X^- + 2 CNR$$

This reaction takes place in alcoholic solution.

The dinitrosyldiisocyanoiron compounds are beautifully crystalline substances, of colours varying from orange to dark red. They are stable in the solid state if kept in an open container; in a stoppered one an autocatalytic decomposition occurs. These compounds are soluble in polar organic solvents and are diamagnetic. The dipole moments of the p-tolyl and p-chlorophenyl isocyanide derivatives have been measured in benzene solution and are rather high (about 6 D)[55].

The only available infrared data were recorded for $Fe(NO)_2$-$(CNC_6H_5)_2$[35]. The values of the NO stretching frequency (1730 and 1707 cm^{-1}) are rather similar to those recorded for $Fe(NO)_2(Ph_3P)_2$ (1719 and 1667 cm^{-1}) and are in agreement with the similar π-accepting properties of the two ligands. Comparison with the NO stretching frequencies of $Fe(NO)_2(CO)_2$ (1810 and 1766 cm^{-1}) shows again that the π-accepting ability of the isocyanide is lower than that of carbon monoxide.

Derivatives of dihalotetracarbonyliron (II)

The substitution reaction of diiodotetracarbonyliron (II) was studied by Hieber and coworkers[50b] and later by Horrocks[34], who extended the study to the chloro- and bromo- compounds and used infrared techniques.

The monosubstituted compounds were prepared according to either of the following reactions[34]:

$$Fe(CO)_4(CNR) + X_2 \xrightarrow{ether} Fe(CO)_3(CNR)X_2 + CO \qquad (X = Cl,Br,I) \quad (1)$$

$$Fe(CO)_4I_2 + CNR \xrightarrow{ether} Fe(CO)_3(CNR)I_2 + CO \qquad (2)$$

the same isomer being formed in both cases when $X = I$.

The disubstituted compounds were prepared by reaction 1, starting with $Fe(CO)_3(CNR)_2$. The iodide was prepared by reaction 2 with the stoichiometric quantity of iodine and was the same as in the first case.

The trisubstituted compounds were prepared by method 2, while the tetrasubstituted ones were made from iron (II) salts and isocyanides (see p. 105); with the exception of the tetrasubstituted compounds, the complexes are not very stable, so that it was not always possible to obtain good analyses. However, they are more stable than the starting $Fe(CO)_4X_2$. They are yellow or brown crystalline substances, soluble in organic solvents.

The problem of assigning their steric configuration was solved by use of infrared techniques. The structures are[34]:

L = CO, RNC;   L = RNC.

The appearance of a weak CN stretching band in addition to those required by the symmetry in $Fe(CO)_2(t\text{-}BuNC)_2I_2$ was attributed either to steric repulsion between the bulky t-butyl group and iodine with consequent distortion of the molecule or to the smaller inductive effect of the iodine as compared to the chlorine with the following higher back-donation and distortion of the Fe—C—NR angle from 180°C.

The thermal decomposition which liberates RNC was found to be very pH and temperature sensitive. It was followed by the change of electronic spectra, in the presence of 1,10-phenanthnoline. The rate was found to be first order toward both the complex and the hydroxyl concentration. The values calculated for the activation energy and the activation entropy were 20·2 Kcal and −1·6 entropy unit/mole respectively.

Mössbauer spectra are available for some of these compounds and are given in Table 6.6[57]. A simple treatment predicts a quadrupole splitting ratio *trans*:*cis* of 2:1, as found here.

RUTHENIUM

The isocyanide compounds of ruthenium so far prepared[58,59] are all derivatives of Ru^{II} with the general formula $RuX_2(CNR)_4$ ($X = Cl, Br, I, CN; R = $ alkyl and aryl) (Malatesta and coworkers). Like the analogous iron compounds, they are all diamagnetic.

The dichloro and dibromo derivatives were prepared[58] by boiling in alcohol a mixture of $RuCl_3$ or $RuBr_3$ and an excess of alkyl or aryl isocyanide. The reaction can be written as follows:

$$RuCl_3 + 4\,RNC + e^- \rightarrow RuCl_2(CNR)_4 + Cl^-$$

The reducing agent may be either the solvent or an excess of the isocyanide itself. On cooling the alcoholic solution, the products separated in a crystalline state. The diiodo and dicyano derivatives[59] could not be obtained in this way probably because of the polymeric structure of RuI_3 and $Ru(CN)_3$.

The iodo compounds were prepared from the diiododicarbonyl-ruthenium (II), $RuI_2(CO)_2$, by warming it with pure aryl isocyanide. From the reaction mixture the product was obtained by extracting it with hot alcohol. No well-defined compounds with alkyl iso-cyanides have been obtained by this method.

The compounds $RuX_2(CNR)_4$ ($X = $ halogen) occur in two forms of different colours and solubilities, which in some cases could not be separated. Both forms are non-electrolytes and monomeric in solution, and it seems likely that they are the *cis-trans* isomers of dihalogeno-tetrakis(isocyanide)ruthenium (II).

The dicyanide derivatives were prepared either by treating the corresponding chloro and bromo compounds with silver cyanide, in chloroform suspension, or by alkylation of hexacyanoruthenic (II) acid, $H_4[Ru(CN)_6]$. The first method gave satisfactory results only with compounds containing alkyl isocyanides. The alkylation re-action was carried out with diazomethane according to a method proposed by Meyer[60,61], both on the free hexacyanoruthenic (II) acid in anhydrous ether and on its etherate in ethyl ether. In the first case a compound of formula $Ru(CN)_2(CNCH_3)_4$ was obtained which was identical with that prepared from $RuBr_2(CNCH_3)_4$ with AgCN; in the other case a compound, $Ru(CN)(OH)(CNCH_3)_4$, was isolated which can be considered a hydrolysis product of the dicyano derivative.

Using diphenyldiazomethane, $(C_6H_5)_2CN_2$, instead of diazo-methane, the compound $Ru(CN)_2[CN.CH(C_6H_5)_2]_4$ was obtained.

This derives from the diphenylmethylisocyanide, which has not been isolated in the free state. It is remarkable that all these dicyano derivatives have been obtained in only one form, usually colourless crystals, soluble in chloroform, very sparingly soluble in alcohol.

On treating with bromine and iodine, the compounds RuX_2-$(CNR)_4$ give crystalline products of dark colours, probably poly-bromides and polyiodides, which, on boiling in solution, are reconverted into the starting compounds.

A similar $Ru(p\text{-}CH_3OC_6H_4NC)_4I$ compound was prepared by prolonged reaction of $Ru(CO)_2(C_5H_5N)I_2$ in benzene at 80° and was found to contain clathrated benzene. The same benzene-containing compound was obtained similarly from $Ru(CO)_2I_2$. Crystallization from acetone ether gave the solvent-free compound as an oil, which crystallized on standing[62].

Table 6.1 Isocyanide derivatives of iron without CO, NO or C_5H_5 groups

Name	Formula	M.p. °C	Colour	Other data	Ref.
a) Complexes with an (apparent) coordination number < 6					
Dichlorobis(n-amyl isocyanide)iron (II)	$FeCl_2(CNC_5H_{11})_2$	—	Golden yellow		33
Dichlorobis(isoamyl isocyanide)iron (II)	$FeCl_2(CNC_5H_{11})_2$	—	Golden yellow		33
Dichlorobis(phenyl isocyanide)iron (II)	$FeCl_2(CNC_6H_5)_2$	—	Golden yellow		33
Bis(isoamyl isocyanide)iron (II) sulphate	$Fe(CNC_5H_{11})_2SO_4$	—	Intense yellow		33
Tetrakis(phenyl isocyanide)iron (II) perchlorate	$[Fe(CNC_6H_5)_4](ClO_4)_2$	—	Yellow needles		37
Tetrakis(o-tolyl isocyanide)iron (II) perchlorate	$[Fe(CNC_7H_7)_4](ClO_4)_2$	—	Yellow needles		37
Tetrakis(p-tolyl isocyanide)iron (II) perchlorate	$[Fe(CNC_7H_7)_4](ClO_4)_2$	—	Yellow needles	$\Lambda_\infty = 42$ ohm^{-1} cm^{-2} ($C_6H_5NO_2$, 20°)	37
Tetrakis(p-chlorophenyl isocyanide)iron (II) perchlorate	$[Fe(CNC_6H_4Cl)_4](ClO_4)_2$	—	Yellow needles		37
b) Complexes with six isocyanide ligands					
Hexakis(methyl isocyanide)iron (II) chloride trihydrate	$[Fe(CNCH_3)_6]Cl_2 . 3\ H_2O$	—	Faintly yellow prisms	$\lambda = 263$ (ε 340) and λ 315 (ε 320) Λ_0:112·5 ohm^{-1} cm^2 (25°) ν(CN):2234vs, 2197w	9, 26, 27, 28, 63
The same, anhydrous	$[Fe(CNCH_3)_6]Cl_2$	—	—	Thermogravimetric analysis	27
Hexakis(methyl isocyanide)iron (II) dibromide, dihydrate	$[Fe(CNCH_3)_6]Br_2 . 2\ H_2O$	196–198	—	ν(CN):2234vs, 2197w (nujol) ν(CN):2238s (KBr)	8
Hexakis(methyl isocyanide)iron(II) iodide, adduct with silver iodide	$[Fe(CNCH_3)_6]I . 4\ AgI$	—	Grey		10
Hexakis(methyl isocyanide)iron (II) nitrate	$[Fe(CNCH_3)_6](NO_3)_2$	—	White crystals		10
Hexakis(methyl isocyanide)iron (II) hydrogen sulphate	$[Fe(CNCH_3)_6](HSO_4)_2$	220 dec.	White crystals	Mössbauer spectrum	6
Hexakis(methyl isocyanide)iron (II) methylsulphate	$[Fe(CNCH_3)_6](CH_3SO_4)_2$	—	White crystals	Very hygroscopic	31
Hexakis(methyl isocyanide)iron (II) methylsulphate with methylsulphuric acid	$[Fe(CNCH_3)_6](CH_3SO_4)_2 . 2\ CH_3HSO_4$	—	White crystals		6

Hexakis(methyl isocyanide)iron (II) hexachloroplatinate	[Fe(CNCH₃)₆]PtCl₆	White small crystals	—	—	31
Hexakis(methyl isocyanide)iron (II) triiodide	[Fe(CNCH₃)₆](I₃)₂	Dark shining crystals	—	—	10
Hexakis(ethyl isocyanide)iron (II) diperchlorate	[Fe(CNC₂H₅)₆](ClO₄)₂	Colourless	—	Mössbauer spectrum	6
Hexakis(benzyl isocyanide)iron (II) dibromide dihydrate	[Fe(CNC₇H₇)₆]Br₂ . 2 H₂O	—	119–121	—	19
Hexakis(benzyl isocyanide)iron (II) diperchlorate	[Fe(CNC₇H₇)₆](ClO₄)₂	—	163·5-164	ν(CN):2212vs (CHCl₃) Electrical conductivity of the solid Mössbauer spectrum	19, 25, 57

c) Complexes of Fe^II with five isocyanide groups

Pentakis(methyl isocyanide)cyanoiron iodide, hydrate	[Fe(CNCH₃)₅CN]I . H₂O	—	137–139	ν(CN):2215s, 2140m (KBr) Λ(C₆H₅NO₂), 0·001 M, 25°): 2·67 × 10⁻⁵ ohm⁻¹ cm⁻¹	8
Pentakis(ethyl isocyanide)cyanoiron triiodide	[Fe(CNC₂H₅)₅CN]I₃	—	109–110·5	Unsuitable for Mössbauer spectrum λ = 27,000 cm⁻¹	57
Pentakis(allyl isocyanide)cyanoiron bromide, hydrated	[Fe(CNC₃H₅)₅CN]Br . H₂O	—	56–58	—	19
Pentakis(3-phenoxypropyl isocyanide)-cyanoiron bromide, hydrated	[Fe(CNC₉H₁₁O)₅CN]Br . H₂O	—	—	ν(CN):2208vs, 2113s, (CHCl₃)	21
Pentakis(12-isocyanododecanoic acid)-bromoiron bromide, trihydrate	[Fe(CNC₁₂H₂₃O₂)₅Br]Br . 3 H₂O	—	61–63	ν(CN):2222 (CHCl₃)	21
Pentakis(n-hexadecyl isocyanide)-cyanoiron iodide	[Fe(CNC₁₆H₃₃)₅CN]I	—	229–231·5	ν(CN):2197vs, 2118s (CHCl₃)	21
Pentakis(benzyl isocyanide)cyanoiron chloride, dihydrated	[Fe(CNC₇H₇)₅CN]Cl . 2 H₂O	—	106–108·5	—	19, 22
Pentakis(benzyl isocyanide)cyanoiron bromide, hydrated	[Fe(CNC₇H₇)₅CN]Br . 2 H₂O	Yellowish needle	101–104	ν(CN):2192 and 2120; ν(OH):3330 (CHCl₃) X-ray diffraction data	8, 19
The same, anhydrous	[Fe(CNC₇H₇)₅CN]Br	—	111–112	(C₆H₅NO₂, 0·001 M, 25°): 2·58 × 10⁻⁵ ohm⁻¹ cm⁻¹. χ = −0·48 × 10⁻⁵ c.g.s.; n.m.r. spectrum. Electrical conductivity of the solid	19, 24, 25
The same, iodide, hydrated (?)	[Fe(C₇H₇)₅CN]I . 2 H₂O	—	119·2–119·6	—	19
The same, thiocyanate	[Fe(CNC₇H₇)₅CN]SCN	—	110–111·2	ν(CN):2165vs, 2118s; 2052s (CHCl₃)	19

Table 6.1 (*continued*)

Name	Formula	Colour	M.p. °C	Other data	Ref.
The same, perchlorate	$[Fe(CNC_7H_7)_5CN]ClO_4$	—	139–140	Electrical conductivity of the solid Mössbauer spectrum	19, 25, 57
The same, hydroxide, pentahydrated	$[Fe(CNC_7H_7)_5CN]OH.5\ H_2O$	—	114·5–117		19
The same, trifluoroacetate	$[Fe(CNC_7H_7)_5CN]COOCF_3$	—	113–115		19
The same, sulphate, dihydrated	$[Fe(CNC_7H_7)_5CN]_2SO_4.2\ H_2O$	—	122–124		19
The same, hydrogensulphate, hydrated	$[Fe(CNC_7H_7)_5CN]HSO_4.H_2O$	—	156·8–157·8	$\nu(CN):2198vs, 2120s\ (CHCl_3)$ Electrical conductivity of the solid	19, 25
The same, nitrate	$[Fe(CNC_7H_7)_5CN]NO_3$	—	106–108	$\nu(CN):2162vs, 2090m\ (CHCl_3)$	19
The same, nitrate, hydrate	$[Fe(CNC_7H_7)_5CN]NO_3.H_2O$	—	85·5–87·5		19
Pentakis(o-methylbenzyl isocyanide)-cyanoiron bromide	$[Fe(CNC_8H_9)_5CN]Br$	—	143·4–145·6	$\nu(CN):2190, 2120\ (CHCl_3)$ n.m.r. spectrum	19, 24, 57
Pentakis(m-methylbenzyl isocyanide)-cyanoiron bromide, hydrate	$[Fe(CNC_8H_9)_5CN]Br.H_2O$	—	oil	$\nu(CN):2190, 2125\ (CHCl_3)$ n.m.r. spectrum	19, 24
Pentakis(p-methylbenzyl isocyanide)-cyanoiron bromide, hydrate	$[Fe(CNC_8H_9)_5CN]Br.H_2O$	—	147·8–149·8	$\chi = -0.32 \times 10^{-5}$c.g. s. $\gamma(CN):2190, 2115\ (CHCl_3)$ n.m.r. spectrum	19, 21
Pentakis(p-chlorobenzyl isocyanide)-cyanoiron bromide	$[Fe(CNC_7H_6Cl)_5CN]Br$	—	160–162·6	$\nu(CN):2189vs, 2125m\ (CHCl_3)$ n.m.r. spectrum	19, 24
Pentakis(p-carbethoxybenzyl isocyanide)-cyanoiron bromide, hydrate	$[Fe(CNC_9H_{11}O_2)_5CN]Br$	—	185–186·2	—	19
Pentakis(p-carbomethoxybenzyl isocyanide)cyanoiron bromide	$[Fe(CNC_9H_9O_2)_5CN]Br$	—	234–237·5	$\nu(CN):2207, 2168; 2068\ (CHCl_3)$ n.m.r. spectrum	21, 24
Pentakis(p-isocyanobenzylsulphonic acid)-cyanoiron hydrogensulphate, trihydrate	$[Fe(CNC_7H_4SO_3)_5CN]$ $HSO_4.3\ H_2O$	—	87–110	$\nu(CN):2212vs, 2118w\ (KBr)$	22
The same, potassium salt	$[Fe(CNC_7H_4KO_3S)_5CN]_2$ $SO_4.2\ H_2O$	—	—	—	22
Pentakis(phenyl isocyanide) bromoiron bromide	$[Fe(CNC_6H_5O)_5Br]Br$	—	219–220	$\nu(CN):2112s, 2173vs\ (KBr)$	21
Pentakis(triphenylmethyl isocyanide)-cyanoiron bromide	$[Fe(CNC_{19}H_{15})_5CN]Br$	—	298–300	—	19
Pentakis(3-bromothenyl isocyanide)-bromoiron bromide, hydrate (?)	$[Fe(CNC_5H_5S)_5Br]Br.H_2O$	—	oil	—	19

Compound	Formula	Colour	M.p.	i.r. spectrum	Ref.
Tetrakis(n-hexadecyl isocyanide)(benzyl isocyanide)cyanoiron iodide	[Fe(CNC₁₆H₃₃)₄(CNC₇H₇)CN]I	—	90·5–93	ν(CN):2188vs, 2128 (CHCl₃)	21
Tetrakis(p-carbomethoxybenzyl isocyanide)(benzyl isocyanide)cyanoiron bromide, hydrate	[Fe(CNC₉H₉O₂)₄(CNC₇H₇)CN]Br . H₂O	—	123–126	ν(CN):2248vs, 2120s (KBr) ν(OH):3430	21
Tetrakis(p-carbomethoxybenzyl isocyanide)(benzyl isocyanide)cyanoiron bromide	[Fe(CNC₉H₉O₂)₄(CNC₇H₇)CN]Br	—	226–230	ν(CN):2192vs, 2160s (KBr)	21
Tetrakis(p-methylbenzyl isocyanide)-(benzyl isocyanide)cyanoiron bromide	[Fe(CNC₈H₉)₄(CNC₇H₇)CN]Br	—	136–136·5	ν(CN):2192vs, 2123s (KBr)	21
(p-Bromobenzyl isocyanide)tetrakis(benzyl isocyanide)cyanoiron bromide, hydrate	[Fe(CNC₇H₆Br)(CNC₇H₇)₄CN]Br . H₂O	Yellow	oil		22
Tetrakis(p-nitrobenzyl isocyanide)(dinitro-benzyl isocyanide)cyanoiron nitrate, hexahydrate	[Fe(CNC₇H₆NO₂)₄(CNC₇H₅N₂O₄)CN]NO₃ . 6H₂O	Yellow	oil	ν(CN):2208vs, 2128s (KBr)	22
(p-Nitrobenzyl isocyanide)tetrakis(benzyl isocyanide)cyanoiron hydrogen sulphate, hydrate	[Fe(CNC₇H₆NO₂)(CNC₇H₇)₄-CN]HSO₄.H₂O	—	oil		22
The same		Yellow	117–118	Same i.r. spectrum	22
Tetrakis(p-nitrobenzyl isocyanide)(benzyl isocyanide)bromoiron bromide dihydrate	[Fe(CNC₇H₆NO₂)₄(CNC₇H₇)-Br]Br₂H₂O	—	85–88	ν(CN):2202vs, 2118w (KBr) (uncertain structure)	21
Tetrakis(2-naphthylmethyl isocyanide)-(benzyl isocyanide)cyanoiron bromide, hydrate	[Fe(CNC₁₁H₉)₄(CNC₇H₇)CN]-Br . H₂O	—	165–166	ν(CN):2198vs, 2118s (KBr)	21
Tris(p-isopropylbenzyl isocyanide)bis-(diisopropylbenzyl isocyanide)cyanoiron hydrogensulphate	[Fe(CNC₁₀H₁₃)₃⁻(CNC₁₃H₁₉)₂CN] HSO₄	Slightly yellow	oil	ν(CN):2430w, 2182w, 2123s (CHCl₃)	22
Bis(p-nitrobenzyl isocyanide)tris(benzyl isocyanide)cyanoiron hydrogensulphate, trihydrate	[Fe(CNC₇H₆NO₂)₂(CNC₇H₇)₃CN]HSO₄3 H₂O	—	oil		22
Tris(p-carbomethoxybenzyl isocyanide)bis(benzyl isocyanide)cyanoiron bromide	[Fe(CNC₉H₉O₂)₃(CNC₇H₇)₂CN]Br	—	141–142·5	ν(CN(:2248vs; 2120vs (KBr)	22
Bis(p-nitrobenzyl isocyanide)tris(benzyl isocyanide)cyanoiron bromide, hydrate	[Fe(CNC₇H₆NO₂)₂(CNC₇H₇)₃CN]Br . H₂O	—	139–143	ν(CN):2182vs, 2118s (KBr)	21
Bis(2-naphthylmethyl isocyanide)tris-(benzyl isocyanide)cyanoiron bromide, hydrate	[Fe(CNC₁₁H₉)₃(CNC₇H₇)₃CN]Br . H₂O	—	216–218	ν(CN):2112vs, 2188vs, 2118s (KBr)	21

Table 6.1 (continued)

d) Complexes with four isocyanide ligands

Name	Formula	Colour	M.p. °C	Other data	Ref.
Dibromotetrakis(methyl isocyanide)iron	$FeBr_2(CNCH_3)_4$	Brown	—	—	32
Diiodotetrakis(methyl isocyanide)iron	$FeI_2(CNCH_3)_4$	Brown; Yellow	—	—	32
Dicyanotetrakis(methyl isocyanide)iron (*cis* and *trans*)	$Fe(CN)_2(CNCH_3)_4$	Yellow; white	255–257	Yellow tablets with $CHCl_3$ from chloroform. Needles from hot methanol. $\nu(CN)$:2100, 2192 KBr, (*trans*) Mössbauer spectrum. White hexahydrate from water	7,8 12,14 15,57
Dicyanotetrakis(ethyl isocyanide)iron (*cis* and *trans*)	$Fe(CN)_2(CNC_2H_5)_4$	Colourless prisms	212–214 or 203–206 dec.	$\nu(CN)$:2180s, 2100w ($CHCl_3$) Mössbauer spectrum	4, 5, 57
Dicyanotetrakis(n-propyl isocyanide)iron	$Fe(CN)_2(CNC_3H_7)_2$	Colourless needles	100–107 dec.	—	15
Tetrakis(methyl isocyanide)bis(ethyl isocyanide)iron iodide, adduct with mercuric iodide	$[Fe(CNCH_3)_4(CNC_2H_5)_2]I_2 . 2\ HgI_2$	α: bright yellow β: pale yellow	—	—	} 11
cis-tetrakis(t-butyl isocyanide)dichloroiron	$Fe(CNC_4H_9)_4Cl_2$	Yellow	181–184	$\nu(CN)$:2207·2m, 2170·4vs, 2154·0s ($CHCl_3$)	34
cis-Tetrakis(t-butyl isocyanide)dibromoiron	$Fe(CNC_4H_9)_4Br_2$	Reddish-brown	151–155	$\nu(CN)$:2172vs, broad ($CHCl_3$)	34
cis-Tetrakis(p-butyl isocyanide)diiodoiron	$Fe(CNC_4H_9)_4I_2$	Dark-brown	111–115	$\nu(CN)$:2198·1vw, 2173·1vs, broad ($CHCl_3$)	34
trans-Tetrakis(phenyl isocyanide)dichloroiron	$Fe(CNC_6H_5)_4Cl_2$	Violet	—	$\nu(CN)$:2140 ($CHCl_3$)	35
cis-Tetrakis(phenyl isocyanide)dichloroiron	$Fe(CNC_6H_5)_4Cl_2$	Orange	—	$\nu(CN)$:2190m, 2160vs, 2150vs, 2125s ($CHCl_3$)	35
trans-Tetrakis(p-tolyl isocyanide)dichloroiron	$Fe(CNC_7H_7)_4Cl_2$	Blue(EtOH)	—	—	32
cis-Tetrakis(p-tolylisocyanide)dichloroiron	$Fe(CNC_7H_7)_4Cl_2$	Yellow-brown (warm $CHCl_3$)	ca. 130 dec.	(CN):2195·0w, 2159·6s, 2152·0s, 2132·2m ($CHCl_3$)	32, 34
The same, adduct with mercuric chloride	$FeCl_2(CNC_7H_7)_4 . HgCl_2$	Red	—	—	32

Name	Formula	Colour	m.p. (°C)	Notes	Ref.
The same, adduct with mercuric bromide	$FeCl_2(CNC_7H_7)_4 \cdot HgBr_2$	Brick-red	—	—	32
The same, adduct with mercuric iodide	$FeCl_2(CNC_7H_7)_4 \cdot HgI_2$	Deep red	—	—	32
Dibromotetrakis(p-tolyl isocyanide)iron (cis and trans)	$FeBr_2(CNC_7H_7)_4$	Deep blue (cold alcohol)	—	—	32
		Brown (warm chloroform)	200 dec.	$\nu(CN)$:2189·7w, 2152·2vs, 2142·2s, 2131·6m	32, 34
The same, adduct with mercuric iodide	$FeBr_2(CNC_7H_7)_4 \cdot HgI_2$	Brown-red	—	—	32
Diiodotetrakis(p-tolyl isocyanide)iron (cis and trans)	$FeI_2(CNC_7H_7)_4$	Emerald-green prisms (cold alcohol)	—	—	32, 34
Dithiocyanatotetrakis(p-tolyl isocyanide)-iron (cis and trans)	$Fe(SCN)_2(CNC_7H_7)_4$	Brown (warm chloroform); Pale yellow (cold alcohol); Brick-red (warm alcohol)	198–201	$\nu(CN)$:2178·4m, 2130·1vs, broad	32
Dicyanotetrakis(p-chlorophenyl isocyanide)iron (cis and trans)	$Fe(CN)_2(CNC_6H_4Cl)_4$	White crystals (cold alcohol)	—	—	32
cis-Tetrakis(p-chlorophenyl isocyanide)-dichloroiron	$Fe(CNC_6H_4Cl)_4Cl_2$	Pale-yellow crystals; Orange	—	$\nu(CN)$:2190m, 2160vs, 2150vs, 2125s (CHCl$_3$)	35
Tetrakis(p-isocyanobenzylsulphonic acid)-dicyanoiron, adduct with sulphuric acid	$Fe(CNC_7H_7O_3S)_4(CN)_2 \cdot H_2SO_4$	—	152–154	$\nu(CN)$:2172vs, 2100s (KBr)	22
Potassium dichlorotetrakis(p-isocyano-benzensulphonate)ferrate (π)	$K_4[FeCl_2(CNC_6H_4SO_3)_4]$	—	—	—	36
Potassium dibromotetrakis(p-isocyano-benzensulphonate)ferrate (π)	$K_4[FeBr_2(CNC_6H_4SO_3)_4]$	Yellow	—	—	36
Potassium diiodotetrakis(p-isocyano-benzensulphonate)ferrate (π)	$K_4[FeI_2(CNC_6H_4SO_3)_4]$	Light-green	—	—	36
Tetrakis(diphenylmethyl isocyanide)-dicyanoiron	$Fe(CNC_{13}H_{11})_4(CN)_2$	—	242–244	Electrical conductivity of the solid	19, 25
Tetrakis(diphenylmethyl isocyanide)-cyanobromoiron	$Fe(CNC_{13}H_{11})_4(CN)Br$	—	122–123·5	—	19
trans-tetrakis(benzylisocyanide)dicyanoiron	$Fe(CNC_7H_7)_4(CN)_2$	—	229·5–230	$\nu(CN)$:2180, 2092 (CHCl$_3$). Monomer; $\chi = -0.39 \times 10^{-5}$ c.g.s. Raman and n.m.r. spectrum. Electrical conductivity of the solid	8, 19 24, 25
Tetrakis(o-methylbenzyl isocyanide)-dicyanoiron, dihydrate	$Fe(CNC_8H_9)_4(CN)_2 \cdot 2H_2O$	—	247–249·5	—	19

Table 6.1 (*continued*)

Name	Formula	Colour	M.p. °C	Other data	Ref.
The same, anhydrous	$Fe(CNC_8H_9)_4(CN)_2$	—	235–237	$\nu(CN):2223$ (CHCl$_3$) n.m.r. spectrum	24
Tetrakis(diisopropylbenzyl isocyanide)-dicyanoiron, hydrate	$[Fe(CNC_{13}H_{19})_4(CN)_2].H_2O$	—	247–248	$\nu(CN):2392s, 2180vs, 2092s$ (CHCl$_3$)	22
Bis(p-nitrobenzyl isocyanide)bis(dinitrobenzyl isocyanide)dicyanoiron, hydrate	$[Fe(CNC_7H_6NO_2)_2(CNC_7H_5N_2O_4)_2(CN)_2].H_2O$	Yellow	143–144	$\nu(CN):2183vs, 2110s$ (CHCl$_3$)	22
e) Complexes with one isocyanide ligand					
Dihydrogen pentacyano(methyl isocyanide)ferrate (II)	$H_2[Fe(CN)_5(CNCH_3)]$	—	—		15
Dihydrogen pentacyano(ethyl isocyanide)ferrate (II)	$H_2[Fe(CN)_5(CNC_2H_5)]$	—	—		15
Aquodicyanotris(methyl isocyanide)iron	$Fe(H_2O)(CN)_2(CNCH_3)_3$	Red	—		7
f) Complexes of Fe^{III}					
Trichlorobis(ethyl isocyanide)iron (III)	$FeCl_3(C_2H_5NC)_2$	Yellow prisms	—		30
Trichlorotris(ethyl isocyanide)iron (III)	$FeCl_3(CNC_2H_5)_3$	Green-yellow leaflets	—		30
Oxotetrachlorotetrakis(ethyl isocyanide)-diiron (III)	$Fe_2Cl_4O(CNC_2H_5/4)$	Yellow square tablets	—		30
Oxotetrachloropentakis(ethyl isocyanide)-diiron (III)	$Fe_2Cl_4O(CNC_2H_5)_5$	Golden-yellow	—		30
Tetrakis(triphenylmethyl isocyanide)-dicyanoiron (III) bromide	$[Fe(CNC_{19}H_{15})_4(CN)_2]Br$	—	303–306·5	$\chi = +1\cdot46 \times 10^{-6}$ c.g.s. (26°C) Electrical conductivity of the solid	15, 25

Table 6.2 Cyclopentadienyl and cyclopentadienylcarbonyl isocyanide complexes of iron

Compound	Formula	Colour	M.p. °C	Infrared data	Conductivity and other data	Ref.
Cyclopentadienylcarbonyl(phenyl isocyanide)iodoiron (II)	$C_5H_5Fe(CO)(CNC_6H_5)I$	Brown Black	108 89	KI:2151, 1969, 2137, 2058, 2000	—	38–39
Cyclopentadienylbis(phenyl isocyanide)-iodoiron (II)	$C_5H_5Fe(CNC_6H_5)_2I$	Red	104–105	KI:2155s, 2096s, 2024w	—	38
Cyclopentadienylbis(phenyl isocyanide)-bromoiron (II)	$C_5H_5Fe(CNC_6H_5)_2Br$	Purple	107	KI:2155s, 2087s, 2020w	—	38
Cyclopentadienyltris(phenyl isocyanide)-iron (II) chloride	$C_5H_5Fe(CNC_6H_5)_3Cl$	Orange	174	KCl:2190, 2123	$\Lambda(25°,\ C_6H_5NO_2)$:28·4	38
Cyclopentadienylcarbonylbis(methyl isocyanide)iron (II) iodide	$C_5H_5Fe(CO)(CNCH_3)_2I$	Yellow	220–221 dec.	KBr:2000 (CO), 2200 (CN)	$\Lambda(23°,\ H_2O,\ 10^{-3}M)$:91 $\Lambda(23°,\ C_6H_5NO_2,\ 2\times10^{-4}M)$:28·1	40
Cyclopentadienylcarbonylbis(allyl isocyanide)iron (II) bromide	$C_5H_5Fe(CO)(CNC_3H_5)_2Br$	Yellow-brown	110–113	KBr:2010 (CO), 2200 (CN)	Powerful CNR odour	40
Cyclopentadienylcarbonylbis(benzyl isocyanide)iron (II) bromide	$C_5H_5Fe(CO)(CNC_7H_7)_2Br$	Golden-yellow	132–133·5	KBr:2010 (CO), 2200 (CN)	$\Lambda(23°,\ H_2O,\ 10^{-3}M)$:89·7 $\Lambda(23°,\ C_6H_5NO_2,\ 2\times10^{-4}M)$:24·6	40
Cyclopentadienylcarbonyl(p-carbethoxy-benzyl isocyanide)iron (II)	$C_5H_5Fe(CO)(CNC_{10}H_{11}O_2)$	Mustard-yellow	166–166·5	KBr:1975 (CO), 2105 (CN), 2200 (CNR)	C_6H_5 and carbonyl absorptions in the i.r.	40
Cyclopentadienylcarbonyl(p-carboxybenzyl isocyanide)cyanoiron (II)	$C_5H_5Fe(CO)(CNC_8H_7O_2)CN$	Yellow	167·5–168·5	KBr:1990 (CO), 2100 (CN), 2180 (CNR)	Infrared evidence for the acid	40
Cyclopentadienylcarbonyl(p-chlorobenzyl isocyanide)cyanoiron (II)	$C_5H_5Fe(CO)(CNC_7H_6Cl)CN$	Yellow	113–115	KBr:2000 (CO), 2115 (CN), 2205 (CNR)	—	40
Cyclopentadienylcarbonyl(triphenylmethyl isocyanide)cyanoiron (II)	$C_5H_5Fe(CO)(CNC_{19}H_{15})CN$	Yellow-brown	181–183 dec.	KBr:1990 (CO), 2090 (CN), 2140 (CNR)	—	40
Cyclopentadienylcarbonyl(benzyl isocyanide)cyanoiron (II)	$C_5H_5Fe(CO)(CNC_7H_7)CN$	Brown oil	—	Film:1970 (CO), 2090 (CN), 2170 (CNR)	—	40
Cyclopentadienylcarbonyl(allyl isocyanide)-cyanoiron (II)	$C_5H_5Fe(CO)(CNC_3H_5)CN$	Brown oil	—	Film:1980 (CO), 2100 (CN), 2185 (CNR)	—	40
μ-carbonyl-μ-phenyl isocyanidebis(cyclopentadienylcarbonyliron)	$(C_5H_5)_2Fe_2(CO)_3(CNC_6H_5)$	—	—	KI:2400, 1949, 1795, 1704 (CNR)	X-ray structure	42
Bis[carbonylcyclopentadienyl(phenyl isocyanide)iron]	$[(C_5H_5)Fe(CNC_6H_5)]_2$	—	—		—	42

Table 6.3 Carbonyl isocyanide complexes of iron (o)

Name	Formula	Colour	M.p. °C	I.r. data	Other data	Ref.
Tetracarbonyl[(methyl isocyanide)iron (o)	Fe(CO)$_4$(CNCH$_3$)	Pale yellow	31·5	CHCl$_3$:2213; 2059 1993, 1961	Dipole moment (5·07D)	44, 51, 52
Tetracarbonyl[(ethyl isocyanide)-iron (o)	Fe(CO)$_4$(CNC$_2$H$_5$)	Pale yellow	−3	CHCl$_3$:2059·1(A$_1$), 1993·4(A$_1$), 1996·6(E)	v(CN) not reported	44, 63
Tetracarbonyl[(t-butyl isocyanide)iron (o)	Fe(CO)$_4$(CNC$_4$H$_9$)	Yellow	53·5-54·5; 48-49	CHCl$_3$:2183; 2057, 1992, 1964		34, 50, 52
Tetracarbonyl[(phenyl isocyanide)iron (o)	Fe(CO)$_4$(CNC$_6$H$_5$)	Pale yellow	60·5-61	CHCl$_3$:2165; 2054, 1994, 1970		34, 44, 51
Tetracarbonyl[(p-tolyl isocyanide)iron (o)	Fe(CO)$_4$(CNC$_7$H$_7$)	Light yellow	50-52		Subl. at 75°/0.001	34
Tetracarbonyl[(p-anisyl isocyanide)iron (o)	Fe(CO)$_4$(CNC$_7$H$_7$O)	Yellow needles	39-40			44
Bis(tetracarbonyl)(1,4-phenylenediisocyanide)iron (o)	Fe$_2$(CO)$_8$[(CN)$_2$C$_6$H$_4$]	Yellow crystals	dec. > 100			44
Tetracarbonyl[(trimethylsilyl isocyanide)iron (o)	Fe(CO)$_4$(CNC$_3$H$_9$Si)	Yellow needles	47-48	CHCl$_3$:2132; 2050, 1996, 1972	Easily sublimed	45, 51
Tetracarbonyl[(trimethylgermyl isocyanide)iron (o)	Fe(CO)$_4$(CNC$_3$H$_9$Ge)	Light yellow	69-70	CHCl$_3$:2135; 2057, 1997, 1968	Subl. at 45°/0·5	45, 51
Tetracarbonyl[(trimethylstannyl isocyanide)iron (o)	Fe(CO)$_4$(CNC$_3$H$_9$Sn)	Light yellow	—	CHCl$_3$:2142; 2065, 2002, 1986	Subl. at 110-115/0·2	45, 51
Tricarbonylbis(methyl isocyanide)iron (o)	Fe(CO)$_3$(CNCH$_3$)$_2$	Colourless leaflets	100-130 dec.	CHCl$_3$:2170; 2009w, 1925		44, 51
Tricarbonylbis(ethyl isocyanide)iron (o)	Fe(CO)$_3$(CNC$_2$H$_5$)$_2$	Pale yellow	65·5-66·5	CHCl$_3$:2155; 2004w, 1922		44, 51
Tricarbonylbis(t-butyl isocyanide)iron (o)	Fe(CO)$_3$(CNC$_4$H$_9$)$_2$	Yellow needles	98-98·5, 92-93	CHCl$_3$:2199, 2090vw; 1944w, 1919		34,51, 52
Tricarbonylbis(p-tolyl isocyanide)iron (o)	Fe(CO)$_3$(CNC$_7$H$_7$)$_2$	Yellow	101-103	—		34
Tricarbonylbis(p-anisyl isocyanide)iron (o)	Fe(CO)$_3$(CNC$_7$H$_7$O)$_2$	Yellow	89-91·5	—		44
Tricarbonyl[(methyl isocyanide) (ethyl isocyanide)iron (o)	Fe(CO)$_3$(CNC$_2$H$_5$)(CNCH$_3$)	Yellow	dec. > 60	—	Needles from P. ether Tablets from MeOH	44

Table 6.4 Nitrosyl isocyanide complexes of iron

Name	Formula	Colour	dec. p.	Ref.
Dinitrosylbis(methyl isocyanide)iron	$Fe(NO)_2(CNCH_3)_2$	Red-brown needles	150–200	50
Dinitrosylbis(ethyl isocyanide)iron	$Fe(NO)_2(CNC_2H_5)_2$	Red–brown needles	97–97·5 (sharp, m.p.)	50
Dinitrosylbis(phenyl isocyanide)iron	$Fe(NO)_2(CNC_6H_5)_2$	Red–brown needles[a]	140–143	50
Dinitrosylbis(p-tolyl isocyanide)iron	$Fe(NO)_2(CNC_7H_7)_2$	Brick-red needles	180–182	55
Dinitrosylbis(p-anisyl isocyanide)iron	$Fe(NO)_2(CNC_7H_7O)_2$	Red-brown needles	197–199	55
Dinitrosylbis(p-chloro-phenyl isocyanide)iron	$Fe(NO)_2(CNC_6H_7Cl)_2$	Red needles	197–199	55

[a] Infrared data in chloroform: 1810, 1766 (NO); 2105, 2147 (CN)[35].

Table 6.5 Carbonyl isocyanide complexes of dihaloiron (II)

Name	Formula	Colour	Dec. point	ν(CN) in CHCl$_3$[a]	ν(CO) in CHCl$_3$[a]	Ref.
Tricarbonyl(p-tolyl isocyanide)dichloroiron	Fe(CO)$_3$(CNC$_7$H$_7$)Cl$_2$	Yellow	90–92	2215·9vs	2132·5s, 2096·5n, 2070·7m	34
Tricarbonyl(t-butyl isocyanide)dichloroiron	Fe(CO)$_3$(CNC$_4$H$_9$)Cl$_2$	Yellow	—	2227·3vs	2131·0s, 2093·1m, 2068·2m	34
Dicarbonylbis(p-tolyl isocyanide)dichloroiron	Fe(CO$_2$)(CNC$_7$H$_7$)$_2$Cl$_2$	Yellow brown	~95	2194·4vs, 2162·5m	2068·8m, 2047·8m	34
Dicarbonylbis(t-butyl isocyanide)dichloroiron	Fe(CO)$_2$(CNC$_4$H$_9$)$_2$Cl$_2$	Yellow	180–185	2207·1vs	2082·1m, 2039·8m	34
Carbonyltris(p-tolyl isocyanide)dichloroiron	Fe(CO)(CNC$_7$H$_7$)$_3$Cl$_2$	Yellow	95–100	2188·0sh, 2173·7vs, 2166·8vs	2037·6m	34
Tricarbonyl(p-tolyl isocyanide)dibromoiron	Fe(CO)$_3$(CNC$_7$H$_7$)Br$_2$	Reddish brown	92–95	2209·6vs	2120·8s, 2088·0m, 2063·4m	34
Tricarbonyl(t-butyl isocyanide)dibromoiron	Fe(CO)$_3$(CNC$_4$H$_9$)Br$_2$	Reddish orange	90–95	2222·9vs	2120·1s, 2084·8m, 2059·8m	34
Dicarbonylbis(p-tolyl isocyanide)dibromoiron	Fe(CO)$_2$(CNC$_7$H$_7$)$_2$Br$_2$	Dark brown	90–95	2185·3s, 2170·5m, sh	2080·0m, 2042·5m	34
Dicarbonylbis(t-butyl isocyanide)dibromoiron	Fe(CO)$_2$(CNC$_4$H$_9$)$_2$Br$_2$	Yellow brown	95–98	2198·6vs	2075·4m, 2035·2m	34
Carbonyltris(p-tolyl isocyanide)dibromoiron	Fe(CO)(CNC$_7$H$_7$)$_3$Br$_2$	Yellow orange	ca. 175	2185·0w, sh, 2170·3vs, 2143·3vs	2035·4m	34
Tricarbonyl(methyl isocyanide)diiodoiron	Fe(CO)$_3$(CNCH$_3$)I$_2$	Brown-red cubes Pleochroic prismatic needles	115	—	—	50
Tricarbonyl(p-tolyl isocyanide)diiodoiron	Fe(CO)$_3$(CNC$_7$H$_7$)I$_2$	Brown black	98–100	2197·1vs	2103·0s, 2071·4m, 2049·4m	34, 50
Tricarbonyl(t-butyl isocyanide)diiodoiron	Fe(CO)$_3$(CNC$_4$H$_9$)I$_2$	Light brown	70–74	2208·2vs	2101·6s, 2068·2m, 2047·5m	34, 50
Dicarbonylbis(methyl isocyanide)diiodoiron	Fe(CO)$_2$(CNCH$_3$)$_2$I$_2$	Dark brown	130	—	—	50
Dicarbonylbis(p-tolyl isocyanide)diiodoiron	Fe(CO)$_2$(CNC$_7$H$_7$)$_2$I$_2$	Reddish brown	113–115	2188·4m, 2166·8s	2073·7m, 2039·2m	34
Dicarbonylbis(t-butyl isocyanide)diiodoiron	Fe(CO)$_2$(CNC$_4$H$_9$)$_2$I$_2$	Light brown	108–111	2201·8m, 2179·7vs	2068·9m, 2030·9m	34
Carbonyltris(p-tolyl isocyanide)diiodoiron	Fe(CO)(CNC$_7$H$_7$)$_3$I$_2$	Reddish brown	80–85	2180·0sh, 2166·2vs	2031·7m	34
Carbonyltris(p-tolyl isocyanide)diiodoiron	Fe(CO)(CNC$_7$H$_7$O)$_3$I$_2$	Red brown prisms and needles	>140	—	—	50

[a] The bands assignments can be found in reference (34).

Table 6.6 Mössbauer spectra of isocyanide complexes of iron[57]

Compound	Quadrupole Splitting[a]	Somer Shift[a,b]
[Fe(CNMe)$_6$]HSO$_4$	0·00	−0·02
cis-Fe(CNMe)$_4$(CN)$_2$	0·24	0·00
trans-Fe(CNMe)$_4$(CN)$_2$	0·44	0·00
[Fe(CNEt)$_6$](ClO$_4$)$_2$	0·00	0·00
[Fe(CN)(CNEt)$_5$]ClO$_4$	0·17	+0·04
cis-Fe(CNEt)$_4$(CN)$_2$	0·29	+0·05
trans-Fe(CNEt)$_4$(CN)$_2$	0·59	+0·05
[Fe(CNCH$_2$Ph)$_6$](ClO$_4$)$_2$	0·00	−0·04
[FeCN(CNCH$_2$Ph)$_5$]ClO$_4$	0·28	−0·02
trans-[Fe(CN)$_2$(CNCH$_2$Ph)$_4$]	0·56	−0·01

[a] ±0·05 mm/sec.
[b] Relative to stainless steel

Table 6.7 Isocyanide compounds of ruthenium

Name	Formula	Colour and crystal form	M.p. or dec. temp., °C	Ref.
Dichlorotetrakis(methyl isocyanide)ruthenium (II)	$RuCl_2(CNCH_3)_4$	Grey crystals from isopropyl ether	—	59
Dibromotetrakis(methyl isocyanide)ruthenium (II)	$RuBr_2(CNCH_3)_4$	Yellow-green crystals from cold alcohol; Red and yellow prisms (not separated)	—	59
Dicyanotetrakis(methyl isocyanide)ruthenium (II)	$Ru(CN)_2(CNCH_3)_4$	White crystals	—	59
Hydroxocyanotetrakis(methyl isocyanide)ruthenium (II)	$Ru(CN)(OH)(CNCH_3)_4$	Pale yellow star-like crystals	—	59
Dichlorotetrakis(ethyl isocyanide)ruthenium (II)	$RuCl_2(CNC_2H_5)_4$	Light blue crystals from cold alcohol; Yellow crystals from ethyl ether	—	58
Dibromotetrakis(ethyl isocyanide)ruthenium (II)	$RuBr_2(CNC_2H_5)_4$	Golden-yellow crystals from cold alcohol; Brick-red crystals from isopropyl ether	—	59
Diiodotetrakis(p-anisyl isocyanide)ruthenium (II)·4/3 C_6H_6 with clathrated benzene	$RuI_2(CNC_7H_7O)_4\cdot4/3\ C_6H_6$	Lemon yellow	—	62
Diiodotetrakis(p-anisyl isocyanide)ruthenium (II)	$RuI_2(CNC_7H_7O)_4$	Yellow	(Diam. at 270 and 17°K)	62
Dicyanotetrakis(ethyl isocyanide)ruthenium (II)	$Ru(CN)_2(CNC_2H_5)_4$	White crystals	—	59
Dichlorotetrakis(p-tolyl isocyanide)ruthenium (II)	$RuCl_2(CNC_7H_7)_4$	Green prisms; Yellow prisms from acetone	256 (dec.)	58
Dibromotetrakis(p-tolyl isocyanide)ruthenium (II)	$RuBr_2(CNC_7H_7)_4$	Dark green octahedral crystals	266 (dec.)	58
Diiodotetrakis(p-tolyl isocyanide)ruthenium (II)	$RuI_2(CNC_7H_7)_4$	Colourless crystals	—	59
Dicyanotetrakis(diphenylmethyl isocyanide)ruthenium (II)	$Ru(CN)_2(CNC_{13}H_{11})_4$	Colourless crystals	—	59
Dichlorodiiodotetrakis(p-tolyl isocyanide)ruthenium (II)	$RuCl_2I_2(CNC_7H_7)_4$	Red crystals	159 (dec.)	58
Chlorotriiodotetrakis(p-tolyl isocyanide)ruthenium (II)	$RuClI_3(CNC_7H_7)_4$	Red crystals	159 (dec.)	58
Dibromoenneaniodotetrakis-(p-tolyl isocyanide)ruthenium (II)	$RuBr_2I_9(CNC_7H_7)_4$	Black-green prisms	—	58

REFERENCES

1. E. G. J. Hartley, *J. Chem. Soc.*, **99**, 1549 (1911).
2. H. L. Buff, *Ann. Chem. Pharm.*, **91**, 253 (1854).
3. A. Von Baeyer and V. Villiger, *Chem. Ber.*, **35**, 1201 (1902).
4. M. Freund, *Chem. Ber.*, **21**, 931 (1888).
5. W. Z. Heldt, *J. Org. Chem.*, **26**, 3226 (1961).
6. E. G. J. Hartley, *J. Chem. Soc.*, **97**, 1066 (1910).
7. F. Hoelzl, W. Hauser and M. Eckmann, *Monatsh.*, **48**, 71 (1927).
8. S. C. Malhotra, *J. Inorg. Nucl. Chem.*, **25**, 971 (1963).
9. H. M. Powell and G. W. R. Bartindale, *J. Chem. Soc.*, **1945**, 799.
10. E. G. J. Hartley, *J. Chem. Soc.*, **101**, 705 (1912).
11. E. G. J. Hartley and H. M. Powell, *J. Chem. Soc.*, **1933**, 101.
12. E. G. J. Hartley, *J. Chem. Soc.*, **103**, 1195 (1913).
13. S. Glasstone, *J. Chem. Soc.*, **1930**, 321.
14. H. M. Powell and G. B. Stanger, *J. Chem. Soc.*, **1939**, 1105.
15. J. Meyer, H. Domann and W. Mueller, *Z. anorg. Chem.*, **230**, 336 (1937).
16. *U.S. Patent*, 3,085,103; *Chem. Abstr.*, **59**, 10127e (1964).
17. *U.S. Patent*, 3,062,855; *Chem. Abstr.*, **58**, 9146h (1963).
18. W. Z. Heldt, *Adv. Chem. Ser.*, **37**, 99 (1963).
19. W. Z. Heldt, *J. Inorg. Nucl. Chem.*, **22**, 305 (1961).
20. W. Z. Heldt, *J. Inorg. Nucl. Chem.*, **24**, 73 (1962).
21. W. Z. Heldt, *J. Inorg. Nucl. Chem.*, **24**, 265 (1962).
22. W. Z. Heldt, *J. Org. Chem.*, **27**, 2604 (1962).
23. W. Z. Heldt, *J. Org. Chem.*, **27**, 2608 (1962).
24. W. Z. Heldt, *Inorg. Chem.*, **2**, 1048 (1963).
25. W. Z. Heldt and C. D. Weis, *J. Phys. Chem.*, **67**, 1392 (1963).
26. F. Cappellina and V. Lorenzelli, *Ann. Chim. (Italy)*, **48**, 855 (1958).
27. G. Fabbri and F. Cappellina, *Ann. Chim. (Italy)*, **48**, 909 (1958).
28. V. Carassiti, G. Condorelli and L. L. Condorelli-Costanzo, *Ann. Chim. (Italy)*, **55**, 329 (1965).
29. V. Carassiti and V. Balzani, *Ann. Chim. (Italy)*, **50**, 782 (1960).
30. K. A. Hofmann and G. Bugge, *Chem. Ber.*, **40**, 3759 (1907).
31. E. G. J. Hartley, *J. Chem. Soc.*, **97**, 1725 (1910).
32. L. Malatesta, A. Sacco and G. Padoa, *Ann. Chim. (Italy)*, **43**, 617(1953).
33. L. Malatesta, *Gazz. Chim. Ital.*, **77**, 240 (1947).
34. R. Craig Taylor and W. Horrocks, Jr., *Inorg. Chem.*, **3**, 584 (1964).
35. F. Canziani, F. Cariati and U. Sartorelli, *Ist. Lomb. (Rend. Sc.)* **A98**, 564 (1964).
36. A. Sacco and O. Coletti, *Atti Accad. naz. Lincei, Rend. Classe Sci. fis. mat. nat.*, VIII, **15**, 89 (1953).
37. G. Padoa, *Ann. Chim. (Italy)*, **45**, 28 (1955).
38. K. K. Joshi, P. L. Pauson and W. H. Stubbs, *J. Organomet. chem.*, **1**, 51 (1963).
39. P. L. Pauson and W. H. Stubbs; *Angew Chem.*, **74**, 466 (1962); *Angew Chem. (Int. Edit.)*, **1** (1962).
40. C. E. Coffey, *J. Inorg. Nucl. Chem.*, **25**, 179 (1963).
41. R. B. King, *Inorg. Chem.*, **6**, 25 (1967).
42. K. K. Joshi, O. S. Mills, P. L. Pauson, B. W. Shaw and W. H. Stubbs, *Chem. Comm.*, **1965**, 181.
43. F. Klages and K. Moenkemeyer, *Chem. Ber.*, **83**, 501 (1950).

5*

44. W. Hieber and D. von Pigenot, *Chem. Ber.*, **89**, 193 (1956).
45. D. Seyferth and N. Kahlen, *J. Am. Chem. Soc.*, **82**, 1080 (1960).
46. T. A. Manuel, *Inorg. Chem.*, **3**, 1703 (1964).
47. D. Seyferth and N. Kahlen, *J. Org. Chem.*, **25**, 809 (1960).
48. H. Ulrich, B. Tucker and A. A. R. Sayigh, *Tetrahedron Letters*, **1967**, 731.
49. R. V. G. Ewens and M. W. Lister, *Trans. Farad. Soc.*, **35**, 681 (1959).
50. W. Hieber and D. von Pigenot, *Chem. Ber.*, **89**, 610 (1956).
51. F. A. Cotton and R. V. Parish, *J. Chem. Soc.*, **1960**, 1440.
52. F. A. Cotton and F. Zingales, *J. Am. Chem. Soc.*, **83**, 351 (1961).
53. W. Hieber and E. Weiss, *Z. anorg. Chem.*, **287**, 223 (1956).
54. L. Malatesta and A. Sacco, *Atti Accad. naz. Lincei, Rend. Classe Sci. fis. mat. nat.*, *VIII*, **13**, 264 (1952).
55. L. Malatesta and A. Sacco, *Z. anorg. Chem.*, **273**, 341 (1953).
56. R. Nast and E. Proeschel, *Z. anorg. Chem.*, **256**, 159 (1948).
57. R. R. Berrett and B. W. Fitzsimmons, *J. Chem. Soc.*, *Part A*, **1967**, 525.
58. L. Malatesta, G. Padoa and A. Sonz, *Gazz. Chim. Ital.*, **85**, 1112 (1955).
59. L. Malatesta and G. Padoa, *Ist. Lombardo (Rend. Sc.)*, *Part I*, **91**, 227 (1957).
60. J. Meyer and W. Hinke, *Z. anorg. Chem.*, **204**, 29 (1932).
61. J. Meyer and W. Sporrmann, *Z. anorg. Chem.*, **228**, 341 (1936).
62. W. Hieber and H. Heusinger, *J. Inorg. Nucl. Chem.*, **4**, 179 (1957).
63. A. Reckziegel and M. Bigorgne, *J. Organometal. Chem.*, **3**, 341 (1965).

7 ISOCYANIDE COMPLEXES OF COBALT, RHODIUM AND IRIDIUM

Isocyanide derivatives are known for all the three elements. While derivatives of cobalt in the $+3$, $+2$, $+1$ and (formally) -1 oxidation state are known, only monovalent iridium and rhodium and trivalent rhodium derivatives are known. The coordination number of the cobalt derivatives may be 4, 5 and 6, while for the iridium derivatives only 4 is yet known. Rhodium and iridium derivatives have not been the objects of as many physicochemical investigations as the more interesting cobalt derivatives.

COBALT

Derivatives of cobalt (III)

Compounds obtained by alkylation of hexacyanocobaltates (III)

The alkylation reaction was carried out by Hartley[1] by gently warming a mixture of silver hexacyanocobaltate (III) and methyl iodide. The reaction can be written as follows:

$$Ag_3[Co(CN)_6] + 3\ CH_3I \rightarrow (CH_3)_3Co(CN)_6 + 3\ AgI$$

The 'methylcobalticyanide' thus obtained is a mixture of two isomeric forms, α and β, which can be separated owing to their different solubilities in water and alcohol. The solubility in the α form is 0.16% in water at $7°$ and 0.04% in boiling alcohol; the solubility of the β form is 0.44% in water at $7°$ and 1.4% in boiling alcohol. No interpretation of this isomerism is given by the author, but it is obvious that a tricyanotris(methyl isocyanide)cobalt (III) can exist in two isomeric forms:

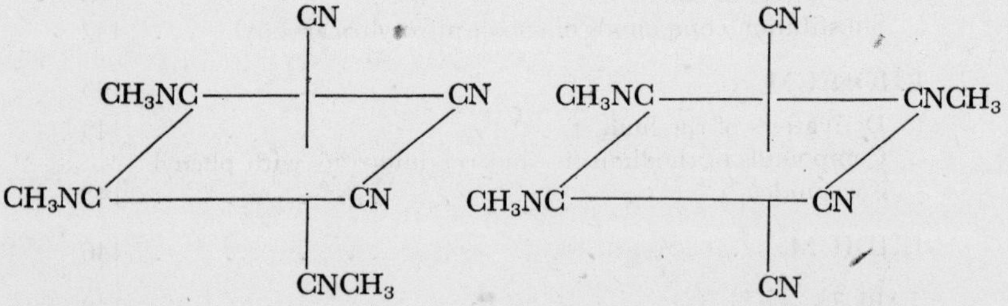

Both the α and the β forms of 'methylcobalticyanide' give insoluble double salts with silver hexacyanocobaltate (III). The formation of these adducts as by-products in the alkylation reaction causes a considerable lowering in the yield of 'methylcobalticyanide'.

Hoelzl and coworkers[2] studied the direct alkylation of hexacyanocobaltic (III) acid with alcohols. The reaction proceeds easily with methanol, with increasing difficulty with ethanol and propanol. Some of the intermediate products were isolated as pyridinium salts, e.g. $(Py)_3H_2[Co(CN)_4(CNCH_3)_2]$ and $(Py)_3H[Co(CN)_5-(CNCH_3)]$. The presence of three pyridine molecules per two and one hydrogen atom, respectively, was not explained by Hoelzl, who called them 'anomalous salts'.

The reaction of $H_3Co(CN)_6$ and alcohol was reinvestigated by Heldt[3] and it is more complex than it would at first appear. An unknown but critical step in the reaction is catalysed by the surface of the autoclave: a new stainless steel autoclave may give only trace yields of the compounds. Previously, the free acid $H_2[Co(CN)_5-(CNC_2H_5)]$ had been obtained by Bolser and Richardson[4].

Other derivatives

Three types of isocyanide derivatives of cobalt (III) have been obtained by reaction of the isocyanide derivatives of cobalt (I) and cobalt (II) with oxidizing agents, such as bromine, iodine, hydrogen peroxide, nitrous acid and amyl nitrite[5]:

(a) The bromides of dibromotetrakis(aryl isocyanide)cobalt (III), $[CoBr_2(CNR)_4]Br$, and the analogous iodo derivatives are well crystallized substances, soluble in chloroform and methylene chloride and insoluble in alcohol. The bromo derivatives are green and the iodo compounds dark brown. These compounds were obtained from the corresponding divalent halides with the required amount of halogen.

(b) The perchlorates of diiodotetrakis(aryl isocyanide)cobalt (III), $[CoI_2(CNR)_4](ClO_4)$, are dark brown crystalline substances, soluble in chloroform with a violet colour. They are obtained either by treating the diiodotetrakis(aryl isocyanide)cobalt (II) compounds with amyl nitrite or hydrogen peroxide, in the presence of perchloric acid, or by addition of the calculated amount of iodine to the perchlorates of pentakis(aryl isocyanide)cobalt (I). It is interesting to note that diiodotetrakis-(benzyl isocyanide)cobalt (II), when oxidized with amyl nitrite or hydrogen peroxide, gives a compound of type (c) instead.

(c) The perchlorates of iodopentakis(aryl isocyanide)cobalt (III), $[CoI(CNR)_5](ClO_4)_2$, are brown-red crystalline substances, soluble in chloroform, insoluble in alcohol. They were prepared from the corresponding perchlorates of pentakis(aryl isocyanide)cobalt (II), on addition of the calculated amount of iodine in methylene chloride.

Compounds of the type $[Co(CNR)_6]^{3+}$ could not be obtained, so that the presence of at least one anionic ligand appears to be essential to the stability of the isocyanide compounds of trivalent cobalt.

> (d) In addition, recent work by Tobe and coworkers[6] showed that the acid-catalysed decomposition of the 4-pyridiomethyl-pentacyanocobaltate (III) ion involved the decomposition of a protonated species, which contains the HNC ligand.

$$\left[\underset{\overset{\oplus}{NH}}{\bigcirc}\!\!-CH_2Co(CN)_5\right]^{3-} \rightleftharpoons \left[\underset{\overset{\oplus}{NH}}{\bigcirc}\!\!-CH_2Co(CN)_4(CNH)\right]^{2-} \longrightarrow$$

$$\left[\underset{\overset{\oplus}{NH}}{\bigcirc}\!\!-CH_2-\underset{\underset{NH}{\parallel}}{C}-Co(CN)_4\right]^{2-}$$

> The same workers also reported that the primary decomposition product was formed by insertion of hydrogen isocyanide into the Co–CH$_2$ bond during the acid-catalysed decomposition of 2-, 3- and 4-pyridiomethylpentacyanocobaltate (III) ions[7].

Derivatives of cobalt (II)

A number of cobalt (II) salts, namely, the halides, the thiocyanate and the perchlorate, react with isocyanides to give addition products of various and interesting types. Most of these compounds are remarkably stable, though less so than the isocyanide derivatives of cobalt (I), into which they can be easily converted by mild reduction. In some cases, for example, with cobalt (II) acetate and nitrate, the reduction to cobalt (I) is spontaneous and immediate, so that the corresponding cobalt (II) compounds cannot be isolated. The isocyanide derivatives of cobalt (III), which can be obtained by oxidation of both Co (I) and Co (II) compounds, are also stable and well-defined substances. Since the cobalt (II) derivatives, when stable, are the first to be obtained in the reaction between cobalt (II) salts and isocyanides, they will be dealt with first.

Cobalt (II) halides form with isocyanides two series of compounds of composition corresponding to $CoX_2(CNR)_2$ and $CoX_2(CNR)_4$. The thiocyanate gives only compounds of the type $Co(SCN)_2(CNR)_2$ and the perchlorate compounds $Co(CNR)_5(ClO_4)_2$.

'Diisocyanide' derivatives

Compounds of formula $CoCl_2(CNCH_3)_2$, $CoBr_2(CNCH_3)_2$ and $Co(SCN)_2(CNCH_3)_2$[5,8] are green crystalline substances, readily soluble in water and methanol, sparingly soluble in organic solvents.

The magnetic susceptibilities of these compounds and also of $[Co(CNCH_3)_4]CdBr_4$ and $[Co(CNCH_3)_4]CdI_4$ were studied thoroughly[9,10]. They allowed formulation of the complex cation $[Co(CNCH_3)_4]^{2+}$ as salts. In the following tabulation, the first column gives the anion, X, present in $[Co(CNCH_3)_4][CoX_4]$; the second, the experimental range of magnetic moment; the third, the value required if the cation were diamagnetic; and the fourth, the value required if a temperature independent magnetic moment of 1·82 BM is assumed for the monomeric cation.

I	II	III	IV
Cl	4·50–4·70	4·94	4·58
Br	4·63–4·77	4·87	4·55
I	4·32–4·40	4·73	4·35

The calculation was carried out on the assumption that the cation had temperature-independent magnetic moment. The θ values (Weiss constants) found were considered to belong to the $[CoX_4]^{2-}$ anion only. The values found for the Weiss constant are in agreement with a possible distortion of the tetrahedral ligand field in $[CoX_4]^{2-}$, owing to bridging by half the X groups, and also with some anti-ferromagnetic coupling between the bridge-connected cationic and anionic Co (II) ions.

The infrared spectrum of $[Co(CNCH_3)_4][Co(SCN)_4]$ shows two CN (from thiocyanato) stretching modes at 2102 and 2072 cm^{-1}; the latter band was assigned to —NCS groups which have free sulphur ends and the former to —NCS groups with sulphur ends coordinated to cationic cobalt (II) atoms.

Reflectance and mull spectra of the compound provide additional support for the original suggestion[8] that the tetrahedral $[CoX_4]^{2-}$ ions are present.

An analogous compound, $CoCl_2(CNC_2H_5)_2$, a green crystalline powder soluble in water and alcohol, had been prepared previously by Hofmann and Bugge[11]. The u.v. absorption spectra of its aqueous solutions[12] had shown that, unlike most addition compounds of this type, it is not decomposed by solvents. However, its structure has not been fully investigated.

The aryl derivative, $CoBr_2(CNC_6H_5)_2$, is a green crystalline powder, insoluble in water and alcohol, and has a magnetic moment near to that of the free Co^{2+} ion[13]. The compounds $Co(SCN)_2$-$(CNAr)_2$ (Ar = phenyl, p-tolyl, p-anisyl) are green crystalline substances, practically insoluble in all solvents, and have magnetic moments like their methyl analogue.

Tetraisocyanide derivatives

The compounds $CoCl_2(CNCH_3)_4$ and $CoBr_2(CNCH_3)_4$[8] are crystalline substances of blue-violet colours, soluble in water, alcohol and nitrobenzene, very sparingly soluble in other organic solvents. The analogous phenyl derivatives, $CoCl_2(CNC_6H_5)_4$ and $CoBr_2(CNC_6H_5)_4$[13], are sparingly soluble crystalline powders.

The isocyanide derivatives of cobalt (II) iodide, described by Malatesta and coworkers[13,14,15], are easily obtained in a pure state by simple addition of isocyanide to an alcoholic solution of cobalt iodide. They have compositions corresponding to $CoI_2(CNR)_4$, where R is alkyl or aryl, and exist in two different forms, called α and β. The compounds of the α-type are diamagnetic crystalline substances, dark green in colour with metallic reflectance when in the form of large crystals, and blue-violet when finely powdered. They are moderately soluble in methylene chloride and nitrobenzene, giving intensely coloured violet solutions, sparingly soluble in the other organic solvents and insoluble in water. The methyl isocyanide derivative is instead a light green crystalline powder, soluble in water and insoluble in organic solvents[8].

The compounds of the β-type are yellow or brown crystalline powders, even less soluble than the corresponding α-forms, and have magnetic susceptibilities corresponding to one unpaired electron.

As the only observed transition in the solid state is $\alpha \rightarrow \beta$, it may be concluded that the β-form is the more stable one. This suggestion is supported by the fact that the α-forms, when they can be obtained, are always the first to separate from the solutions. The α-forms can be transformed into the β by prolonged warming at 40–60°, or more rapidly by boiling in the presence of a solvent in which they are only slightly soluble, e.g. alcohol or acetone. The β-forms, on the other hand, are reconverted into the α by dissolution and reprecipitation from cold solutions. In some cases, a partial $\beta \rightarrow \alpha$ transformation is obtained by finely grinding the β-form. In solution, an equilibrium $\alpha \rightleftharpoons \beta$ is established, which may lie more on one side or the other depending on the solvent and the concentration. Its position can be roughly estimated from the magnetism of the solution. An increase in the concentration always shifts the equilibrium towards the α-form, as may be seen from the fact that the colour of the solution turns from yellow-brown (β-form) to violet (α-form) on concentration.

For the compounds containing aryl isocyanides, the stability of the α-form depends very much on the groups attached to the benzene ring; in some cases the α-form may even become too unstable to be isolated. However, no indication of the reasons for this influence could be inferred from the study of a number of different aryl isocyanide derivatives, nor could any regularity be detected. On the basis of conductivity measurements in dilute solutions, and by analogy with the corresponding chloro and bromo compounds, the β-forms were then considered as tetra(isocyanide)cobalt (II) iodides, $[Co(CNR)_4]I_2$. The diamagnetism of the α-forms might be ascribed either to a resonance of the type Co (I) ↔ Co (III) or to spin pairing between pairs of cobalt (II) atoms. Only an x-ray investigation will make possible an unambiguous assignment of the structure of the α-form. At the moment there are only indirect suggestions, the most substantial of which seems to be the comparison between the α-$CoI_2(CNC_6H_5)_4$ and the analogous diamagnetic rhodium compound, $RhI_2(CNC_6H_5)_4$[16]. In fact, the rhodium compound, for which a dimeric structure, $[Rh_2I_2(CNC_6H_5)_8]I_2$, has been proved on the basis of chemical behaviour, is identical in appearance with the cobalt derivative, and the two compounds have been shown to be isomorphous by comparison of their x-ray powder patterns.

The methyl isocyanide derivative, $CoI_2(CNCH_3)_4$[8] when treated with sodium perchlorate in aqueous solution, gives a compound of composition $Co_2(CNCH_3)_{10}I(ClO_4)_3$, diamagnetic in the solid state, paramagnetic in solution, with a magnetic moment corresponding to one unpaired electron per cobalt atom. To account for the conductivity of its aqueous solutions, this compound was assigned the structure of μ-iododecakis(methyl isocyanide)cobalt (II) perchlorate, $[(CH_3NC)_5CoICo(CNCH_3)_5](ClO_4)_3$. The aryl derivatives, $CoI_2(CNAr)_4$, do not react with sodium perchlorate in chloroform–alcohol solution[14]. With the amount of silver perchlorate exactly calculated to substitute one iodine atom, in chloroform–benzene solution, they give a rather complicated reaction:

$$5 CoI_2(CNAr)_4 + 4 AgClO_4 \rightarrow 4 [CoI(CNAr)_5](ClO_4) + 4 AgI + CoI_2$$

The bromides, $[Co(CNAr)_4]Br_2$, react in an analogous way. The compounds, $[CoX(CNAr)_5](ClO_4)$ (X = Br, I), are black-violet crystalline substances, which in nitrobenzene solution behave as strong uni–univalent electrolytes. In the solid state they are dia-magnetic; no data are available for the magnetic susceptibility of the solutions.

The existence of the cation $[CoX(CNAr)_5]^+$ (X = Br, I)[14] shows that $[Co(CNAr)_5]^{2+}$, though saturated with respect to isocyanides, is not coordinately saturated in the strict sense, as it is able to bind a halogen atom or a water molecule[20].

The diamagnetism of the compounds $[CoX(CNAr)_5](ClO_4)$, even if limited to the solid state, is rather difficult to explain. In fact, since the cobalt atoms are coordinately saturated, it seems difficult to think of a structure where the metal–metal distance would allow spin coupling.

Magnetic and spectral studies were carried out on these violet complexes of methylisocyanide and on the related iodide, tetra-bromo- and tetraiodocadmiate (II). Attempts to prepare the homo-logous compounds with anions less capable or incapable of bridging, e.g. tetraphenylborate or perchlorate, were unsuccessful, the only isolable compounds being derivatives of the pentakisisocyanide-cobalt (II). The coordination of the cobalt atom in the tetraisocy-anide derivatives is more nearly octahedral than planar, owing to halogen bridging. In the CdX_4 compounds, a similar halogen bridg-ing is postulated, this time between Co and Cd atoms. All the magnetic moments found for these complexes lie between 1·82 and 1·89 BM[9]. Preliminary e.s.r. data[17] are now available.

Infrared studies[18] were carried out on the $Co(CNAr)_4X_2$ com-pounds (X = Cl, Br; Ar = phenyl, p-tolyl). A structure with D_{4h} symmetry was assumed because only one i.r. CN stretching vibration was observed in chloroform solution.

Pentaisocyanide derivatives

Compounds having an isocyanide/cobalt (II) ratio of five were first isolated by Sacco[19]. He found that methyl isocyanide afforded two different types of compound, both soluble in water and in alcohol. One is light blue and paramagnetic (one electron spin), the other red and diamagnetic. While in the solid state the latter seems to be the stable one, the solutions are always blue and paramagnetic; they have electric conductivity in agreement with a formula like pentakis-(methyl isocyanide)cobalt (II) perchlorate. The preparation of the blue form of $[Co(CNMe)_5](ClO_4)_2$ could not be repeated by Pratt and Silverman[20]. They suggested that the blue form might have been

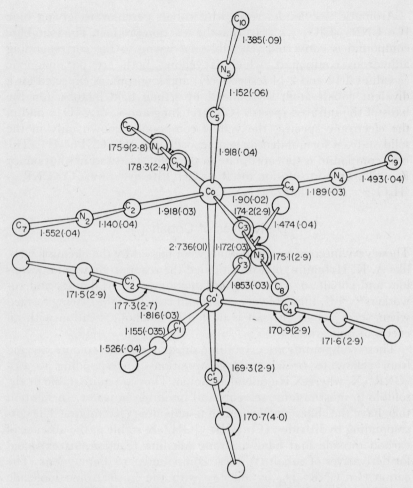

Figure 7.1 Structure and molecular parameters of
[Co$_2$(CNCH$_3$)$_{10}$](ClO$_4$)$_4$

instead a derivative of mauve-coloured [Co(CNMe)$_6$]$^{2+}$. This
latter compound was assumed to be present when an aqueous
solution of pentakis(methyl isocyanide)cobalt (II) perchlorate,
[Co(CNMe)$_5$(H$_2$O)](ClO$_4$)$_2$, was treated with excess methyl
isocyanide. However, the diamagnetism of the red form had been
correctly ascribed to a metal–metal bond, as evidenced by the
structural determination carried out on [Co$_2$(CNMe)$_{10}$](ClO$_4$)$_4$ by
Cotton (Figure 7.1)[21].

Aromatic isocyanides react with cobalt perchlorate, giving blue $[Co(CNR)_5(ClO_4)_2.1\cdot5\,H_2O]$ as the reaction product. The solid blue compound is converted reversibly on drying to the corresponding anhydrous compound, which is yellow; both are paramagnetic (g value: $2\cdot12$ and $2\cdot14$ respectively) and low-spin, as expected for a divalent cobalt atom surrounded by strong field ligands. On the basis of the infrared spectra (CN stretching and ν_3 of ClO_4^-) and of the electronic spectra, the yellow compound, known only in the solid state, is formulated as pentacoordinate, $[Co(CNPh)_5]^{2+}$. The blue compound is six-coordinate in the solid state and in solution for $R = Ph$, only in solution for $R = CH_3$; its structure, $[Co(CNR)_5-(H_2O)^{2+}$, is like that of $[CoX(CNAr)_5]^+$ [14].

Derivatives of Cobalt (I)

These very interesting compounds were missed by the chemists who, like A. K. Hofmann, first investigated the reaction between isocyanides and cobalt (II) salts. Yet, as later shown by Malatesta and co-workers[22,23,24], they are very stable and easy to obtain, being formed whenever a cobalt (II) salt is heated in alcoholic solution with an excess of isocyanide.

These compounds are crystalline substances, with colours varying from yellow to brown, and compositions corresponding to Co-$(CNR)_5X$, where X is a univalent anion. They are quite stable to air, soluble in most organic solvents and insoluble in water. In solution they have the character of strong uni–univalent electrolytes. The corresponding hydroxides, $[Co(CNR)_5]OH$, are stable in the absence of carbon dioxide and have a strong alkaline reaction. As expected for derivatives of cobalt (I), these compounds are diamagnetic. The cation $[Co(CNR)_5]^+$, by analogy with the isoelectronic molecule $Fe(CO)_5$, may be considered to have a trigonal bipyramidal structure. This point was demonstrated by examination of the infrared spectrum in the CN stretching region. Cotton[25] found two i.r. active bands in $[Co(CNPh)_5]ClO_4$ at 2175 (m) and 2120 (s), as required by a trigonal bipyramidal structure; a rectangular pyramidal structure would require three i.r. active CN stretching frequencies.

The molecular parameters of $[Co(CNCH_3)_5]^+$, as determined by Cotton on the perchlorate[26], are given in Figure 7.2.

The most suitable way to prepare the salts of pentaisocyanocobalt (I) is a mild reduction of the divalent derivatives $[Co(CNR)_5]-(ClO_4)_2$ and $Co(CNR)_4I_2$. The pentaisocyanocobalt (II) perchlorates

Bond distances, Å.

Co–C(1)	1.88 ± 0.02
Co–C(5)	1.88 ± 0.02
Co–C(3)	1.84 ± 0.02
C(1)–N(1)	1.14 ± 0.03
C(3)–N(2)	1.14 ± 0.02
C(5)–N(3)	1.15 ± 0.03
N(2)–C(4)	1.44 ± 0.02
N(3)–C(6)	1.44 ± 0.03
N(1)–C(2)	1.45 ± 0.04

Interbond angles, deg.

Co–C(1)–N(1)	180.00
Co–C(3)–N(2)	179 ± 1.3
Co–C(5)–N(3)	180 ± 1.5
C(1)–Co–C(3)	89.2 ± 0.6
C(3)–Co–C(5)	89.3 ± 0.7
C(3)–Co–C(5)′	91.4 ± 0.8
C(1)–Co–C(5)	115.9 ± 0.7
C(5)–Co–C(5)′	128.3 ± 0.8
C(3)–N(2)–C(4)	177 ± 1.5
C(5)–N(3)–C(6)	173 ± 2.0
C(3)–Co–C(3)′	180.00

Intramolecular nonbonded
contact distances, Å.

C(1)–C(3)	2.62 ± 0.03
C(3)–C(5)	2.51 ± 0.03
C(3)–C(5)′	2.66 ± 0.03
C(1)–C(5)	3.19 ± 0.03
C(5)–C(5)′	3.40 ± 0.03

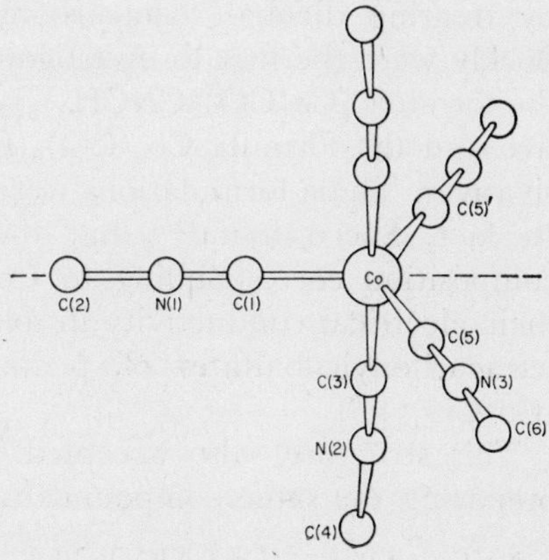

Figure 7.2   Structure and molecular parameters of
$[Co(CNCH_3)_5]ClO_4$

can be reduced by simply boiling them in alcohol in the presence of isocyanide. With hydrazine the reduction takes place immediately in the cold[8]:

$$4\,Co(CNR)_5(ClO_4)_2 + N_2H_4 \rightarrow 4\,Co(CNR)_5ClO_4 + 4\,HClO_4 + N_2$$

The tetraisocyanocobalt (II) iodides require a mild reducing agent, such as dithionite, hydrazine acetate or metals. With hydrazine the reaction proceeds as follows:

$$5\,Co(CNR)_4I_2 + N_2H_4 \rightarrow 4\,Co(CNR)_5I + CoI_2 + 4\,HI + N_2$$

With metals the reaction is analogous and allows isolation of, for example, pentakis(vinyl isocyanide)cobalt (I) nitrate[27]; but, when silver or mercury is used, the final product is an adduct between the pentaisocyanocobalt (I) salt and the silver or mercury salt:

$$5\,Co(CNR)_4I_2 + 4\,Ag \rightarrow 4\,Co(CNR)_5I.AgI + CoI_2$$

$$5\,Co(CNR)_4I_2 + 2\,Hg \rightarrow 2\,\{Co(CNR)_5I\}_2.HgI_2 + CoI_2$$

The addition compounds between the halides of pentaisocyanide-cobalt (I) and the halides of heavy metals can be formulated as halometallates of the cation $[Co(CNR)_5]^+$, e.g. $[Co(CNR)_5]_2 HgI_4$, but it is not possible to formulate in a similar way the analogous addition compounds of $[Co(CNR)_5](ClO_4)$.

The pentakis(aryl isocyanide)cobalt (I) cations are also formed by treating dicobalt octacarbonyl with isocyanides. Hieber and Böckly were the first to investigate this reaction[28]. They attributed the formula $[Co(CO)(CNCH_3)_3]_2$ to the methyl isocyanide derivative and the formula $Co_2(CO)_3(CNR)_5$ to the aryl isocyanide derivatives. These formulations were, however, shown to be incorrect. In fact, Sacco found[29] that the products, when pure, have a composition corresponding to $Co_2(CO)_4(CNR)_5$ and, because of their electrical conductivity in solution, must be formulated as the tetracarbonylcobaltates of pentaisocyanide cobalt $[Co(CNR)_5]-[Co(CO)_4]$[30].

This structure, also accepted by Hieber[30], was confirmed by preparing the same compounds in another way:

$$Na[Co(CO)_4] + [Co(CNR)_5](ClO)_4 \rightarrow [Co(CNR)_5][Co(CO)_4] + NaClO_4$$

The reaction between the dimeric cobalt carbonyl and isocyanides may therefore be written as follows:

$$[Co_2(CO)_8] + 5\ CNR \rightarrow [Co(CNR)_5][Co(CO)_4] + 4\ CO$$

The compound $[Co(CNR)_5][Co(CO)_4]$, which contains one cobalt atom in the $+1$ oxidation state and the other in the -1 oxidation state, can be compared with the product formed by action of ethylenediamine (en) on iron pentacarbonyl, which has the composition $Fe_2(en)_3(CO)_4$[31] and must be formulated as the tetracarbonylferrate (-2) of tris(ethylenediamino)iron$(+2)$, $[Fe(en)_3][Fe(CO)_4]$[32].

The reaction between aryl isocyanides and cobalt carbonyl is indicative of the different abilities of CO and CNR to stabilize the low valent states of the metals. Both ligands, however, tend to give ions where the metal orbitals are completely filled; actually both the pentacoordinated $Co(+1)$ and the tetracoordinated $Co(-1)$ have the effective atomic number of krypton.

Substitution compounds of cobalt nitrosyltricarbonyl

The reaction between $Co(NO)(CO)_3$ and aryl isocyanides takes place rapidly and neatly in alcoholic solution, yielding the nitrosylcarbonyldi(isocyanide)cobalt compounds[33]:

$$[Co(NO)(CO)_3] + 2\ CNR \rightarrow [Co(NO)(CO)(CNR)_2] + 2\ CO$$

Compounds having complete substitution of CNR for CO could not be obtained in this way, but were suitably prepared by treating the black form of nitrosylpentaaminocobalt (II) chloride with isocyanides, in the presence of hydrazine[33]:

$$2 [Co(NO)(NH_3)_5]Cl_2 + 6 CNR + N_2H_4 \rightarrow$$
$$2 Co(NO)(CNR)_3 + N_2 + 6 NH_3 + 4 NH_4Cl$$

The nitrosyltri(alkyl isocyanide)cobalt compounds can also be prepared by reacting the pentaisocyanocobalt (I) salts with hydroxylamine, in alcoholic solution containing ammonia[33,34]. The reaction, analogous to that of iron, was written as follows:

$$2 NH_2OH \rightarrow NH_3 + NOH + H_2O$$
$$[Co(CNR)_5]^+ + NOH + NH_3 \rightarrow Co(NO)(CNR)_3 + NH_4^+ + 2 CNR$$

The nitrosylcarbonylbis(aryl isocyanide)cobalt and nitrosyltris-(aryl isocyanide)cobalt compounds are orange-red crystalline substances, soluble in most organic solvents, quite stable to air. They are all diamagnetic. The nitrosyltris(aryl isocyanide) compounds have rather high dipole moments in benzene solution.

The infrared spectra were studied by Horrocks[35]. According to his data, p-tolyl isocyanide has almost the same π-electron withdrawing ability as diphenylchlorophosphine. In agreement with the accepted inductive effect of alkyl and aryl groups and with results of Bigorgne for nickel and molybdenum carbonylisocyanide compounds, t-butyl isocyanide was found to be slightly less electronegative than tolyl isocyanide.

The influence of the solvent on the infrared CN stretching vibration of $Co(CO)(NO)(CNR)_2$ (R = p-tolyl, t-butyl) was accurately studied by Horrocks[36] (see Table 1.5).

Attempts to prepare other formally Co^{-I} compounds by reaction of bis(tetracarbonylcobaltate)mercury (II) with aliphatic or aromatic isocyanide were unsuccessful: carbon monoxide, mercury and $[CoL_5][Co(CO)_4]$ were the reaction products. On the other hand, the analogous cadmium (II) tetracarbonylcobaltate gave a 1:2 adduct with p-anisyl isocyanide[37].

RHODIUM

Derivatives of rhodium (I)

Rhodium (III) chloride and the other soluble salts and complexes of rhodium (III) do not react with isocyanides in the cold. However, when a solution of rhodium (III) chloride in ethanol is refluxed with an excess of isocyanide, a lively reaction occurs and after many undetermined steps, shown by formation of amorphous precipitates of various colours, a stable blue-violet solution is obtained[40]. On addition of bulky anions, such as ClO_4^- and $[PF_6]^-$, well-crystallized and intensely coloured substances separate from this solution. They are diamagnetic and behave as strong uni–univalent electrolytes. According to their analyses they can be formulated as the salts of tetrakis(aryl isocyanide)rhodium (I), $[Rh(CNR)_4]X$, where X is a univalent anion.

The formation reactions were presumed to be:

$$RhCl_3 + 4\ CNR \rightarrow [RhCl_2(CNR)_4]Cl$$

$$[RhCl_2(CNR)_4]Cl + CNR + H_2O \rightarrow [Rh(CNR)_4]Cl + RNCO + 2\ HCl$$

$$[Rh(CNR)_4]Cl + NaClO_4 \rightarrow [Rh(CNR)_4]ClO_4 + NaCl$$

This is partially confirmed by the isolation of the intermediate trivalent product, $[RhCl_2(CNC_6H_5)_4]Cl$.

The salts of tetrakis(aryl isocyanide)rhodium (I) give stable solvates of different colours and crystal forms with various solvents. This tendency to solvation is quite unusual among the isocyanide complexes and might be explained by postulating that in this case the vacant $5p_z$ orbital of the tetracoordinated rhodium (I) is able to accept a lone electron-pair from a suitable donor molecule. This simple dative bond is much weaker than the isocyanide–metal bonds, and the substitution, as well as the removal, of the molecule of solvent is quite easy. The unsolvated salts can be obtained from benzene, ethyl acetate and alcohols higher than propanol, and are yellow or green; the colours of the solvates vary with the solvent, the anion, and the isocyanide. It must be noted, however, that the proposed explanation does not account for the fact that in some cases two or even more forms, of different colours but having nearly identical compositions, have been obtained for the same solvate.

The salts of tetrakis(aryl isocyanide)rhodium (I) can also be prepared from rhodium carbonyl halides and isocyanides. This method is the more suitable for the preparation of the derivatives of phenyl isocyanide, which are obtained only in very poor yields by the method previously described. When p-anisyl isocyanide is used, the partially substituted intermediate products can be isolated[41]:

$$Rh_2Cl_2(CO)_4 + 4\ CNR \rightarrow 2\ RhCl(CO)(CNR)_2 + 2\ CO$$

$$RhCl(CO)(CNR)_2 + 2\ CNR \rightarrow [Rh(CNR)_4]Cl + CO$$

The chlorocarbonylbis(*p*-anisyl isocyanide)rhodium (I) and the analogous bromo compound are pale-yellow crystalline substances, soluble in chloroform with a red-violet colour. They are non-electrolytes and monomeric in solution. With triphenylphosphine they react giving tetracoordinated salts of rhodium (I)[41]:

$$RhCl(CO)(CNR)_2 + 2\ PR_3 \rightarrow [Rh(CNR)_2(PR_3)_2]Cl + CO$$

An analogous reaction occurs with triarylarsines, triarylstibines and the esters of phosphorous acid. These mixed salts are yellow or orange-yellow crystalline substances, soluble in most organic solvents. Unlike the tetraisocyanide salts, they have no tendency to form solvates.

Compounds of rhodium (II) and rhodium (III) with phenyl isocyanide

It has already been mentioned that the behaviour of phenyl iso-cyanide toward rhodium (III) chloride is somewhat different from that of the other aryl isocyanides. In fact, the blue-violet solution obtained by refluxing phenyl isocyanide and rhodium (III) chloride, under the conditions that usually lead to the univalent tetracoordina-ted salts, yields instead a derivative of trivalent rhodium[16]. This is a diamagnetic, blue-violet crystalline product, which from its analysis and conductivity can be formulated as the chloride of dichloro-tetrakis(phenyl isocyanide)rhodium (III), $[RhCl_2(CNC_6H_5)_4]Cl$. This formulation is confirmed by the formation of the corresponding perchlorate, $[RhCl_2(CNC_6H_5)_4]ClO_4$, on exchange with sodium perchlorate in alcoholic solution. When heated in ethanol in the presence of a slight excess of phenyl isocyanide, this derivative of trivalent rhodium dissolves, giving a red-violet solution from which, on addition of sodium iodide, a dark crystalline product with green reflectances separates[16]. This is a salt-like substance, of analysis corresponding to $RhI_2(CNC_6H_5)_4$. It is diamagnetic both in the solid state and in solution and is strictly similar to the α-form of the corresponding compounds of cobalt (II), (see p. 137), with which it is shown to be isomorphous by comparison of the x-ray powder patterns.

On treating with sodium perchlorate in ethanol, the compound $RhI_2(CNC_6H_5)_4$ gives a dark crystalline substance that can be formulated as the perchlorate of diidooctakis(phenyl isocyanide)-dirhodium (II), $[Rh_2I_2(CNC_6H_5)_8](ClO_4)_2$. This shows that in the iodo compound one of the iodine atoms acts as a ligand and suggests that the compound is the iodide of diiodooctakis(phenyl isocyanide)-dirhodium (II), $[Rh_2I_2(CNC_6H_5)_8]I_2$. On the other hand, when the iodo compound in methylene chloride–alcohol solution is treated with sodium tetraphenylborate, it gives a salt of formula $[Rh_2I_3(CNC_6H_5)_7][B(C_6H_5)_4]$ and a similar product, $[Rh_2I_3(CNC_6H_5)_7]I$, is obtained on reaction with iodine in chloroform solution in the molar ratio 1:1. These facts show that in solutions of chloroform and methylene chloride the equilibrium

$$[Rh_2I_2(CNC_6H_5)_8]I_2 \rightleftharpoons [Rh_2I_3(CNC_6H_5)_7]I + CNC_6H_5$$

is present, which is shifted to the right in the presence of anions capable of forming insoluble salts with univalent cations.

While carbonyl complexes of monovalent rhodium containing aromatic phosphines, arsines and stibines could be oxidized to Rh^{III} compounds, the analogous reaction failed with $Rh(CNPh)_2$-$COCl$ as with $Rh(NH_2R)(CO)_2Cl$[42].

IRIDIUM

No iridium isocyanide complex was known up to 1961. Reaction of polymeric IrX_3 (X = Cl, Br, I) with the ligand was unsuccessful, no addition or reaction product being formed. The use of reducing agents, in the hope of obtaining Ir^I complexes, as with rhodium, was not successful either: a mild reducing agent was ineffective, a strong one gave metallic iridium.

However, Malatesta[45] isolated iridium (I) compounds by the ready reaction of cis-$Ir(CO)_2(p$-toluidine)Cl and p-tolyl isocyanide in methylene chloride at room temperature. Diamagnetic dark green $[Ir(CO)(CNC_7H_7)_3]Cl$ was isolated by precipitation with hexane.

When the reaction was carried out in refluxing methanol, and excess p-tolyl isocyanide was used, a very soluble, deep blue compound was left after evaporation. This residue was converted into more manageable compounds by addition of sodium bromide, iodide or perchlorate to the aqueous solution. The electrolytic conductances of the compounds are in agreement with their formulation as 1:1 electrolytes. No other physical data could be recorded.

It is interesting to compare the series Co^I, Rh^I and Ir^I. Cobalt (I) gives the extremely stable pentacoordinate $[Co(CNR)_5]^+$, rhodium (I) gives tetracoordinated compounds, which however form stable addition products with polar solvents; iridium (I) is apparently tetracoordinate and has no evident reactivity like that of the remarkable tetracoordinate $Ir(CO)_2(PPh_3)Cl$.

Table 7.1 Isocyanide compounds of cobalt

Name	Formula	M.p. °C	Colour	(CN) and other data	Ref.
a) Nitrosyl derivatives					
Nitrosylcarbonylbis(p-tolyl isocyanide)cobalt (−1)	$Co(NO)(CO)(CNC_7H_7)_2$	153–159 (dec.) 133–136	Orange-red needles	C_6H_{12}:2135, 2086; 1987; 1745	33, 34, 35
Nitrosylcarbonylbis(t-butyl isocyanide)cobalt (−1)	$Co(NO)(CO)(CNC_4H_9)_2$	—	Orange-red	C_6H_{12}:2141·8, 2108·4; 1975·5; 1733·3	35, 36
Nitrosyltris(p-tolyl isocyanide)cobalt (−1)	$Co(NO)(CNC_7H_7)_3$	157–160 dec.	Red needles	Dipole moment	33
Nitrosyltris(p-anisyl isocyanide)cobalt (−1)	$Co(NO)(CNC_7H_7O)_3$	130–134 dec.	Orange needles	Dipole moment	33
Nitrosyltris(p-chlorophenyl isocyanide)cobalt (−1)	$Co(NO)(CNC_6H_4Cl)_3$	107–108 dec.	Orange needles	Dipole moment	33
b) Derivatives of Cobalt (i)					
Pentakis(methyl isocyanide)cobalt (i) perchlorate	$[Co(CNCH_3)_5]ClO_4$	—	Yellow needles	Nujol:2140s, 2205m, 2270w	8, 20
Pentakis(methyl isocyanide)cobalt (i) tetracarbonylcobaltate (−1)	$[Co(CNCH_3)_5][Co(CO)_4]$	—	Pale yellow needles	CH_2Cl_2:2152s, 2190m; −96[a]; x-ray structure	26, 28
Pentakis(vinyl isocyanide)cobalt (i) nitrate	$[Co(CNC_2H_3)_5](NO_3)$	114–117 dec.	Brown crystals	2152, 2118	27, 38
Pentakis(vinyl isocyanide)cobalt (i) tetraphenylborate	$[Co(CNC_2H_3)_5]B(C_6H_5)_4$	130	Yellow needles	2152, 2118	27, 38
Pentakis[2-(p-toluensulphonyl)ethyl isocyanide]cobalt (i) tetraphenylborate	$[Co(CNC_9H_{11}O_3S)_5][BC_{24}H_{20}]$	57–63	Brown crystals	2180, 2097	38
Pentakis[2-(p-toluensulphonyl)ethyl isocyanide]cobalt (i) hexafluorophosphate	$[Co(CNC_9H_{11}O_3S)_5][PF_6]$	38	Brown crystals	2180, 2097	38
Pentakis(phenyl isocyanide)cobalt (i) iodide	$[Co(CNC_6H_5)_5]I$	—	Orange prisms	−140[a]	22

The same, adduct with mercuric iodide	Co(CN)(C$_6$H$_5$)$_5$]I.HgI$_2$	Brown leaflets	115 dec.	−249^a	22
Pentakis(phenyl isocyanide)cobalt (I) nitrate	[Co(CNC$_6$H$_5$)$_5$]NO$_3$	Pale yellow	—	—	22
Pentakis(phenyl isocyanide)cobalt (I) chlorate	[Co(CNC$_6$H$_5$)$_5$]ClO$_3$	Pale yellow	—	—	22
Pentakis(phenyl isocyanide)cobalt (I) perchlorate	[Co(CNC$_6$H$_5$)$_5$]ClO$_4$	Yellow needles	—	CH$_2$Cl$_2$:2120s, 2160s CHCl$_3$:2175m, 2120s −320^a	20, 22, 25
Pentakis(o-tolyl isocyanide)cobalt (I) perchlorate	[Co(CNC$_7$H$_7$)$_5$]ClO$_4$	Golden-yellow needles	—	−372^a	22
Adduct of pentakis(p-tolyl isocyanide)-cobalt (I) bromide with mercuric bromide	[Co(CNC$_7$H$_7$)$_5$]Br.HgBr$_2$	Yellow leaflets	155–160 dec.	−210^a	22
Pentakis(p-tolyl isocyanide)cobalt (I) iodide	[Co(CNC$_7$H$_7$)$_5$]I	Orange-red prisms	99–100 dec.	−270^a 17·85^b	22
The same, adduct with mercuric iodide	Co(CNC$_7$H$_7$)$_5$]I.HgI$_2$	Brick-red prisms	120–125 dec.	−289^a	22
The same, adduct with mercurous iodide	[Co(CNC$_7$H$_7$)$_5$]I$_2$.Hg$_2$I$_2$	Golden-yellow needles	110–115 dec.	−590^a	22
The same, adduct with mercurous iodide	Co(CNC$_7$H$_7$)$_5$]I.Hg$_2$I$_2$	Orange prisms	154 dec.	−320^a	22
The same, adduct with silver iodide	Co(CNC$_7$H$_7$)$_5$]I.AgI	Amber coloured crystals	150 dec.	−210^a	22
The same, adduct with cadmium iodide	[Co(CNC$_7$H$_7$)$_5$]I$_2$.CdI$_2$	Tobacco coloured prisms	165–170 dec.	−512^a	22
Pentakis(p-tolyl isocyanide)cobalt (I) perchlorate	[Co(CNC$_7$H$_7$)$_5$]ClO$_4$	Golden-yellow needles	—	−450^a 22·8^c	22
The same, adduct with mercuric iodide	[Co(CNC$_7$H$_7$)$_5$]ClO$_4$.HgI$_2$	Deep red prisms	—	—	22
Pentakis(p-tolyl isocyanide)cobalt (I) tetracarbonylcobaltate (−I)	[Co(CNC$_7$H$_7$)$_5$][Co(CO)$_4$]	Brown-yellow needles	—	—	29
Pentakis(p-chlorophenyl isocyanide)-cobalt (I) iodide	[Co(CNC$_6$H$_4$Cl)$_5$]I	Yellow-orange prisms	—	−30^a	22

^{a} Magnetic susceptibility of the solid at 20°C, × 10^{-6} c.g.s. units.
^{b} Conductivity of 1/5000 M nitrobenzene solution at 19°C.
^{c} Conductivity at 19°C in 0·001 M nitrobenzene solution.

Table 7.1 (*continued*)

Name	Formula	Colour	M.p. °C	ν(CN) and other data	Ref.
Pentakis(*p*-chlorophenyl isocyanide)cobalt(I) nitrate	[Co(CNC$_6$H$_4$Cl)$_5$]NO$_3$	Pale-yellow prisms	—	—	23
Pentakis(*p*-chlorophenyl isocyanide)cobalt(I) chlorate	[Co(CNC$_6$H$_4$Cl)$_5$]ClO$_3$	Pale-yellow prisms	—	—	23
Pentakis(*p*-chlorophenyl isocyanide)cobalt(I) perchlorate	[Co(CNC$_6$H$_4$Cl)$_5$]ClO$_4$	Yellow needles	—	−335[a]	22
Pentakis(*p*-chlorophenyl isocyanide)cobalt(I) tetracarbonylcobaltate(−1)	[Co(CNC$_6$H$_4$Cl)$_5$][Co(CO)$_4$]	Yellow needles	—	—	8
Pentakis(3-chloro-2-methylphenyl isocyanide)cobalt(I) perchlorate	[Co(CNC$_7$H$_6$Cl)$_5$]ClO$_4$	Yellow needles	—	−361[a]	22
Pentakis(β-naphthyl isocyanide)cobalt(I) iodide	[Co(CNC$_{10}$H$_7$)$_5$]I	Yellow-orange prisms	—	—	22
c) Derivatives of Cobalt (II)					
Tetrakis(methyl isocyanide)cobalt(II) tetrachlorocobaltate(II)	[Co(CNCH$_3$)$_4$]CoCl$_4$	Green	220 dec.	8940[a,d]; 524[f]	8, 9
Tetrakis(methylisocyanide)cobalt(II) tetrabromocobaltate(II)	[Co(CNCH$_3$)$_4$]CoBr$_4$	Green	243 dec.	9166[a,d]; 470[f]	8, 9
Tetrakis(methyl isocyanide)cobalt(II) tetrabromocadmiate	[Co(CNCH$_3$)$_4$]CdBr$_4$	Pink	245 dec.	1·82[d,h]	9
Tetrakis(methyl isocyanide)cobalt(II) tetraiodocadmiate	[Co(CNCH$_3$)$_4$]CdI$_4$	Light brown	260	1·82[d,h]	9
Tetrakis(methyl isocyanide)cobalt(II) tetrathiocyanato cobaltate(II)	[Co(CNCH$_3$)$_4$][Co(SCN)$_4$]	Green	158 dec.	7640[a,d]	8
Dichlorobis(ethyl isocyanide)cobalt(II)	CoCl$_2$(CNC$_2$H$_5$)$_2$	Green pleochroic crystals	—	—	11, 12
Dibromobis(phenyl isocyanide)cobalt(II)	CoBr$_2$(CNC$_6$H$_5$)$_2$	Green powder	—	4·47[h]	13
Dichlorotetrakis(methyl isocyanide)cobalt(II)	CoCl$_2$(CNCH$_3$)$_4$	Violet	—	1·89[d,h]	9
Dibromotetrakis(methyl isocyanide)cobalt(II)	CoBr$_2$(CNCH$_3$)$_4$	Violet	—	1·84[d,h]	9

Compound	Formula	m.p. (°C)	Colour	Data	Refs.
Diiodotetrakis(methyl isocyanide)cobalt(II)	$CoI_2(CNCH_3)_4$	—	Olive green powder	−180[a]; 1050[g]	⎫ 8, 9
Iododecakis(methyl isocyanide)dicobalt(II) perchlorate	$[Co_2I(CNCH_3)_{10}](ClO_4)_3$	—	Brown crystals	1160[a]; 245[f]	⎬
Dichlorotetrakis(phenyl isocyanide)cobalt(II)	$CoCl_2(CNC_6H_5)_4$	—	Dark brown crystals	−82[a]; 370[f]; 1100[g]	8
		—	Brown	$CHCl_3$:2190	18
trans-Dibromotetrakis(phenyl isocyanide)cobalt(II)	$CoBr_2(CNC_6H_5)_4$	250 dec.	Violet or green	Nujol: 2210w, 2182 vs; $CHCl_3$:2190; 3·27[h]	13, 18
Diiodotetrakis(phenyl isocyanide)cobalt(II)	$CoI_2(CNC_6H_5)_4$	222 dec.	Green needles	$CHCl_3$:2188; 1·99[h]	13, 18
		—	Dark green or violet	⎰ Nujol:2202w, 2177s; $CHCl_3$:2182; 164[a], 1372[e]	13, 18
		—	Black or brown	⎱ $CHCl_3$:2182; 1440[a]	13, 18
Dibromotetrakis(p-tolyl isocyanide)cobalt(II)	$CoBr_2(CNC_7H_7)_4$	—	Green	$CHCl_3$:2190	18
Diiodotetrakis(p-anisyl isocyanide)cobalt(II)	$CoI_2(CNC_7H_7O)_4$	—	Dark green crystals	−168[a]	⎫ 14
Diiodotetrakis(m-chlorophenyl isocyanide)cobalt(II)	$CoI_2(CNC_6H_4Cl)_4$	—	Brown crystals	6·54[a]; 6·93[i]; 1475[a]	⎬
		—	Yellow-brown	1380[a]	14
Diiodotetrakis(p-chlorophenyl isocyanide)cobalt(II)	$CoI_2(CNC_6H_4Cl)_4$	—	Yellow-brown	1487[a]	14
Diiodotetrakis(2,4-dimethylphenyl isocyanide)cobalt(II)	$CoI_2(CNC_8H_9)_4$	—	Yellow-brown	1400[a]	14
Diiodotetrakis(3-chloro-2-methyl-phenyl isocyanide)cobalt(II)	$CoI_2(CNC_7H_6Cl)_4$	—	Violet crystals	110[a]	14
Diiodotetrakis(4-chloro-2-methyl-phenyl isocyanide)cobalt(II)	$CoI_2(CNC_7H_6Cl)_4$	—	Yellow-brown Yellow-brown	1270[a] 1190[a]	14

[a] Magnetic susceptibilities at different temperatures are known[9].
[e] Magnetic susceptibility in chloroform solution.
[f] Conductivity at 15°C in 0·001 M aqueous solution.
[g] Magnetic susceptibility in aqueous solution at 20°C.
[h] Magnetic moment, B.M. (uncorrected).
[i] Conductivity in 0·0015 M dichloromethane solution at 17°C.

Table 7.1 *(continued)*

Name	Formula	M.p. °C	Colour	(CN) and other data	Ref.
Diiodotetrakis(2,5-dichlorophenyl isocyanide)cobalt(II)	$CoI_2(CNC_6H_3Cl_2)_4$	—	Dark crystals with green reflectance	−80[a]	14
Diiodotetrakis(β-naphthyl isocyanide)cobalt(II)	$CoI_2(CNC_{10}H_7)_4$	—	Brown crystals; Blue powder; Brown powder	1264[a]; −30[a]; 1270[a]	14
Potassium dibromotetrakis(p-isocyanobenzensulphonate)cobaltate(II)	$K_4[CoBr_2(CNC_6H_4SO_3)_2]$	—	Dark brown powder	1198[a]	39
Cobalt(II) dibromotetrakis(p-isocyanobenzoato)cobaltate(II)	$Co_2[CoBr_2(CNC_6H_4COO)_4]$	—	Brown substance	14,025[a]	39
Cobalt(II) diiodotetrakis(p-isocyanobenzoato)cobaltate(II)	$Co_2[CoI_2(CNC_6H_4COO)_4]$	—	Dark blue substance	14,020[a]	39
Bromopentakis(phenyl isocyanide)cobalt(II) perchlorate	$[CoBr(CNC_6H_5)_5]ClO_4$	—	Black crystals	90[a]	14
Iodopentakis(phenyl isocyanide)cobalt(II) perchlorate	$[CoI(CNC_6H_5)_5]ClO_4$	—	Black crystals	80[a]	14
Iodopentakis(p-tolyl isocyanide)cobalt(II) perchlorate	$[CoI(CNC_7H_7)_5]ClO_4$	—	Black crystals		14
Iodopentakis(p-anisyl isocyanide)cobalt(II) perchlorate	$[CoI(CNC_7H_7O)_5]ClO_4$	—	Black crystals	218[f]; 118[a]	14
Pentakis(methyl isocyanide)cobalt(II) perchlorate	$[Co(CNCH_3)_5](ClO_4)_2$	152 dec.	Red crystalline powder	Dimer with Co—Co bond[21] Nujol:2230sh, 2170s −120[a]; 1260[g]	8, 20, 21
		—	Blue crystals	1265[a]	8, 20

Compound	Formula	Description	IR data	Ref
Pentakis(phenyl isocyanide)cobalt (II) perchlorate	$[Co(CNC_6H_5)_5](ClO_4)_2$	Yellow	$\begin{cases} \text{Nujol:}2180, 2220s^k; \\ \text{e.s.r. data} \end{cases}$	20
The same, sesquihydrate	$[Co(CNC_6H_5)_5]$ $(ClO_4)_2.1\cdot5\ H_2O$	Green blue needles	Nujol:2190sh, 2220s;	19, 20
Pentakis(o-tolyl isocyanide)cobalt (II) perchlorate	$[Co(CNC_7H_7)_5](ClO_4)_2$	Green needles	$1270^{a,k}$; e.s.r. data 1293^a	19
Pentakis(p-tolyl isocyanide)cobalt (II) perchlorate	$[Co(CNC_7H_7)_5]$ $(ClO_4)_2$	Green needles	1286^a ; $23\cdot2^c$	19
d) Derivatives of Cobalt (III)				
Dibromotetrakis(phenyl isocyanide)-cobalt (III) bromide	$[CoBr_2(CNC_6H_5)_4]Br$	Dark green prisms	—	5
Diiodotetrakis(p-tolyl isocyanide)-cobalt (III) iodide	$[CoI_2(CNC_7H_7)_4]I$	Dark brown prisms	—	5
Diiodotetrakis(p-anisyl isocyanide)-cobalt (III) iodide	$[CoI_2(CNC_7H_7O)_4]I$	Dark green prisms	—	5
Diiodotetrakis(2-chloro-6-methyl-phenyl isocyanide)cobalt (III) perchlorate	$[CoI_2(CNC_7H_6Cl)_4]ClO_4$	Brown prisms	—	5
Diiodotetrakis(p-tolyl isocyanide)-cobalt (III) perchlorate	$[CoI_2(CNC_7H_7)_4]ClO_4$	Dark brown prisms	—	5
Iodopentakis(o-tolyl isocyanide)-cobalt (III) perchlorate	$[CoI(CNC_7H_7)_5](ClO_4)_2$	Brown prisms	—	5
Iodopentakis(p-tolyl isocyanide)-cobalt (III) perchlorate	$[CoI(CNC_7H_7)_5](ClO_4)_2$	Dark brown prisms	—	5
Iodopentakis(benzyl isocyanide)-cobalt (III) perchlorate	$[CoI(CNC_7H_7)_5](ClO_4)_2$	Red violet tablets	—	5

^{k} Electronic spectra are available[20].

Table 7.2 Isocyanide compounds of rhodium

Name	Formula	Colour and crystal form	M.p. or dec. temp., °C	Other data	Ref.
Chlorocarbonylbis(p-anisyl isocyanide)rhodium (I)	$RhCl(CO)(CNC_7H_7O)_2$	Ivory white needles	140–150 (dec.)	—	41
Bromocarbonylbis(p-anisyl isocyanide)rhodium (I)	$RhBr(CO)(CNC_7H_7O)_2$	Pale yellow needles	165–170	—	41
Tetrakis(phenyl isocyanide)rhodium (I) perchlorate	$[Rh(CNC_6H_5)_4]ClO_4$	Yellow prisms (from benzene)	172–180	—	40
Tetrakis(p-tolyl isocyanide)rhodium (I) perchlorate	$[Rh(CNC_7H_7)_4]ClO_4$	Yellow tablets (from benzene)	198 (dec.)	-50×10^{-6a} 30^b	40
		Violet needles (from ethanol)	207 (dec.)	-60×10^{-6a} 31^b	43, 44
		Blue needles (from methanol)	200 (dec.)	-80×10^{-6a} 31^b	40
Tetrakis(p-anisyl isocyanide)rhodium (I) perchlorate	$[Rh(CNC_7H_7O)_4]ClO_4$	Green needles	180 (dec.)	30^b	
		Green leaflets (from benzene)	230 (dec.)	-90×10^{-6a} 28^b	40
Tetrakis(p-anisyl isocyanide)rhodium (I) hexafluorophosphate	$[Rh(CNC_7H_7O)_4]PF_6$	Bright red needles (from aqueous ethanol)	215 (dec.)	-70×10^{-6a}	
		Violet tablets (from chloroform)	237 (dec.)	-60×10^{-6a}	40
Tetrakis(p-chlorophenyl isocyanide)rhodium (I) chloride	$[Rh(CNC_6H_4Cl)_4]Cl$	Blue hair-like needles (from methanol)	140 (dec.)	-50×10^{-6a}	40
Bis(phenyl isocyanide)bis(triphenylphosphine)rhodium (I) chloride	$[Rh(CNC_6H_5)_2\{(C_6H_5)_3P\}_2]Cl$	Violet prisms (from ethanol) Yellow prisms	137 (dec.) 165–170	-135×10^{-6a}	41 41

Name	Formula	Appearance	M.p.		Ref.
Bis(phenyl isocyanide)bis(triphenylphosphine)rhodium (I) bromide	[Rh(CNC$_6$H$_5$)$_2${(C$_6$H$_5$)$_3$P}$_2$]Br	Yellow prisms	180–185 (dec.)		41
Bis(phenyl isocyanide)bis(triphenylphosphine)rhodium (I) iodide	[Rh(CNC$_6$H$_5$)$_2${(C$_6$H$_5$)$_3$P}$_2$]I	Yellow-brown prisms	180–185 (dec.)		41
Bis(p-anisyl isocyanide)bis-(triphenylphosphine)rhodium(I) chloride	[Rh(CNC$_7$H$_7$O)$_2${(C$_6$H$_5$)$_3$P}$_2$]Cl	Yellow needles	140–145 (dec.)	19·0ᶜ	41
Bis(p-anisyl isocyanide)bis(triphenylphosphine)rhodium (I) iodide	[Rh(CNC$_7$H$_7$O)$_2${(C$_6$H$_5$)$_3$P}$_2$]I	Orange needles	155–160 (dec.)	18·8ᶜ	41
Bis(p-anisyl isocyanide)bis(triphenylphosphine)rhodium (I) perchlorate	[Rh(CNC$_7$H$_7$O)$_2${(C$_6$H$_5$)$_3$P$_2$]ClO$_4$	Yellow prisms	180 (dec.)	20·1ᶜ	41
Bis(p-anisyl isocyanide)bis(triphenylarsine)rhodium (I) perchlorate	[Rh(CNC$_7$H$_7$O)$_2${(C$_6$H$_5$)$_3$As}$_2$]ClO$_4$	Yellow-orange prisms	185–190 (dec.)	19·8ᶜ	41
Bis(p-anisyl isocyanide)bis(triphenylstibine)rhodium (I) perchlorate	[Rh(CNC$_7$H$_7$O)$_2${(C$_6$H$_5$)$_3$Sb}$_2$]ClO$_4$	Yellow prisms	180–190 (dec.)	21·0ᶜ	41
Bis(p-anisyl isocyanide)bis(triphenylphosphite)rhodium (I) perchlorate	[Rh(CNC$_7$H$_7$O)$_2${(C$_6$H$_5$O)$_3$P}$_2$]ClO$_4$	Yellow prisms	157–160 (dec.)	23·9ᶜ	41
Diiodooctakis(phenyl isocyanide)-dirhodium(II) iodide	[Rh$_2$I$_2$(CNC$_6$H$_5$)$_8$]I$_2$	Dark crystals with green reflectances	140–145 (dec.)		16
Diiodooctakis(phenyl isocyanide)-dirhodium(II) perchlorate	[Rh$_2$I$_2$(CNC$_6$H$_5$)$_8$](ClO$_4$)$_2$	Dark leaflets with metallic reflectances	210–215		16
Triiodoheptakis(phenyl isocyanide)-dirhodium(II) tetraphenylborate	[Rh$_2$I$_3$(CNC$_6$H$_5$)$_7$][(C$_6$H$_5$)$_4$B]	Deep red needles	141–142		16
Triiodoheptakis(phenyl isocyanide)-dirhodium(II) triiodide	[Rh$_2$I$_3$(CNC$_6$H$_5$)$_7$]I$_3$	Deep red needles with green reflectances	130–135 (dec.)		16
Dichlorotetrakis(phenyl isocyanide)-rhodium (III) chloride	[RhCl$_2$(CNC$_6$H$_5$)$_4$]Cl	Blue-violet prisms	140–145 (dec.)		16
Dichlorotetrakis(phenyl isocyanide)-rhodium (III) perchlorate	[RhCl$_2$(CNC$_6$H$_5$)$_4$]ClO$_4$	Olive green hair-like needles	210–215 (dec.)		16

ᵃ Magnetic susceptibility of the solid.
ᵇ Molar conductivity in nitrobenzene at infinite dilution.
ᶜ Molar conductivity in 1/1000 M nitrobenzene solution.

Table 7.3   Isocyanide compounds of iridium[a]

Name	Formula	Colour	M.p. °C	Λ in nitrobenzene
Carbonyltris(p-tolyl isocyanide)chloroiridium (I)	$IrCl(CO)(CNC_7H_7)_3$	dark green	250	24 ohm^{-1}cm^2 (10^{-4}molar, 20°C)
Tetrakis(p-tolyl isocyanide)iridium bromide	$[Ir(CNC_7H_7)_4]Br$	blue green	>260 (dec.)	—
Tetrakis(p-tolyl isocyanide)iridium iodide	$[Ir(CNC_7H_7)_4]I$	green	>260 (dec.)	—
Tetrakis(p-tolyl isocyanide)iridium perchlorate	$[Ir(CNC_7H_7)_4]ClO_4$	dark green	>260 (dec.)	27 ohm^{-1}cm^2 (2 × 10^{-4} molar, 20°C

[a] All data from ref. 45.   All the compounds are diamagnetic.

REFERENCES

1. E. G. J. Hartley, *J. Chem. Soc.*, **105**, 521 (1914).
2. F. Hoelzl, T. Meier-Mohar and F. Viditz, *Monatsh.*, **53–54**, 237 (1929).
3. W. Z. Heldt, *J. Org. Chem.*, **26**, 3226 (1961).
4. C. E. Bolser and L. B. Richardson, *J. Am. Chem. Soc.*, **35**, 377 (1913).
5. A. Sacco, *Atti Accad. naz. Lincei, Rend. Classe Sci. fis. mat.*, [*VIII*], **12**, 82 (1953).
6. M. D. Johnson, M. L. Tobe and Lai-Yoong Wong, *Chem. Comm.*, **1967**, 298.
7. M. D. Johnson, M. L. Tobe and Lai-Yoong Wong, *J. Chem. Soc., Part A*, **1967**, 491.
8. A. Sacco and M. Freni, *Angew. Chem.*, **70**, 599 (1957); A. Sacco and M. Freni, *Gazz. Chim. Ital.*, **89**, 1800 (1959).
9. A. Sacco and F. A. Cotton, *J. Am. Chem. Soc.*, **84**, 2043 (1962).
10. F. A. Cotton and R. H. Holm, *J. Am. Chem. Soc.*, **82**, 2983 (1960).
11. K. A. Hofmann and G. Bugge, *Chem. Ber.*, **40**, 3759 (1907).
12. A. Hantzsch, *Z. anorg. Chem.*, **159**, 273 (1927).
13. L. Malatesta and L. Giuffre, *Atti. Accad. naz. Lincei, Rend. Classe Sci. fis. mat. nat.*, [*VIII*], **11**, 206 (1951).
14. L. Malatesta and A. Sacco, *Gazz. Chim. Ital.*, **83**, 499 (1953).
15. L. Malatesta, *Gazz. Chim. Ital.*, **83**, 958 (1953).
16. L. Vallarino, paper presented at the International Conference on Coordination Chemistry, London, 1959.
17. J. P. Maher, *Chem. Comm.*, **1967**, 632.
18. F. Canziani, F. Cariati and U. Sartorelli, *Ist. Lombardo (Rend. Sc.)*, **A98**, 564 (1964).
19. A. Sacco, *Gazz. Chim. Ital.*, **84**, 370 (1954).
20. J. M. Pratt and P. R. Silverman, *Chem. Comm.*, **1967**, 117.
21. F. A. Cotton, T. G. Dunne and J. S. Wood, *Inorg. Chem.*, **3**, 1495 (1964).
22. L. Malatesta and A. Sacco, *Z. anorg. Chem.*, **273**, 247 (1953).
23. L. Malatesta and A. Sacco, *Atti Accad naz. Lincei, Rend. Classe Sci. fis. mat. nat.*, [*VIII*], **13**, 264 (1952).
24. L. Malatesta, unpublished results.
25. F. A. Cotton and R. V. Parish, *J. Chem. Soc.*, **1960**, 1440.

26. F. A. Cotton, T. G. Dunne and J. S. Wood, *Inorg. Chem.*, **4**, 318 (1965).
27. D. S. Matteson and R. A. Bailey, *Chem. and Ind.*, **1967**, 191.
28. W. Hieber and E. Bockly, *Z. anorg. Chem.*, **262**, 344 (1950).
29. A. Sacco, *Gazz. Chim. Ital.*, **83**, 622 (1953).
30. W. Hieber and J. Sedlmeier, *Chem. Ber.*, **89**, 92 (1954).
31. W. Hieber and H. Vetter, *Chem. Ber.*, **64**, 2340 (1931).
32. W. Hieber, R. Nast and J. Sedlmeier, *Angew. Chem.*, **64**, 465 (1952).
33. L. Malatesta and A. Sacco, *Z. anorg. Chem.*, **273**, 341 (1953)
34. L. Malatesta and A. Sacco, *Atti Accad. naz. Lincei, Classe Sci. fis. mat. nat.*, [*VIII*], **13**, 264 (1952).
35. W. D. Horrocks, Jr., R. Craig Taylor, *Inorg. Chem.*, **2**, 723 (1963).
36. W. D. Horrocks, Jr. and R. H. Mann, *Spectrochim. Acta*, **19**, 1375 (1963).
37. W. Hieber and R. Breu, *Chem. Ber.*, **90**, 1259 (1957).
38. D. S. Matteson, personal communication (June 29, 1967).
39. A. Sacco and O. Coletti, *Atti Accad. naz. Lincei, Rend. Classe sci. fis. mat. nat.*, [*VIII*], **15**, 89 (1953).
40. L. Malatesta and L. Vallarino, *J. Chem. Soc.*, **1956**, 1867.
41. L. Vallarino, *Gazz. Chim. Ital.*, **89**, 1632 (1959); L. Vallarino, *Ist. Lombardo (Rend. Sci.), Part I*, **91**, 397 (1957).
42. L. Vallarino, *J. Inorg. Nucl. Chem.*, **8**, 288 (1958); L. Vallarino, *Ist. Lombardo (Rend. Sc.), Part I*, **91**, 399 (1957).
43. L. Vallarino, *J. Chem. Soc.*, **1957**, 2473.
44. L. Vallarino, *J. Chem. Soc.*, **1957**, 2287.
45. L. Malatesta, *U.S. Dept. of Commerce, Office Tech. Serv.*, AD 262,065, 10 (1961); *Chem. Abstr.*, **58**, 4596f (1963).

8 ISOCYANIDE COMPLEXES OF NICKEL, PALLADIUM AND PLATINUM

Very few analogies can be observed among the isocyanide compounds of the elements of this triad. In the divalent state they all form derivatives of the type $MeX_2 . 2\,CNR$; but, while the nickel compounds are often ill defined and unstable, those of palladium and platinum are extensively stable and well characterized, though their physical properties were not studied at the time of their characterization. Besides, palladium compounds exist only in the monomeric nonionic form, $PdX_2(CNR)_2$, while those of platinum were obtained both as $[Pt(CNR)_4][PtX_4]$ and $PtX_2(CNR)_2$.

In the zerovalent state, nickel forms tetracoordinated compounds, $Ni(CNR)_4$, soluble in organic solvents, whereas palladium gives insoluble $Pd(CNR)_2$ compounds. No zerovalent platinum derivative has so far been described.

NICKEL

Derivatives of nickel (II)

A lively and very exothermic reaction occurs on addition of isocyanides to an alcoholic solution of nickel salts, which shows that the affinity of isocyanides towards Ni^{2+} is quite strong. Nevertheless, none of the products obtained by reacting nickel chloride and nickel cyanide with isocyanides is a stable and well-defined substance. They are brown powders that cannot be recrystallized and on heating do not melt sharply but gradually decompose into a black molten mass. Their compositions correspond to the formulae $NiCl_2(CNR)_2$, $Ni(CN)_2(CNR)_2$ and $Ni(CN)_2(CNR)_4$, and they were considered to be isocyanide complexes of divalent nickel[7]. However, their lack of definite properties, together with the observation that they act as catalysts in the polymerization of free isocyanides, makes such a formulation rather doubtful. Indeed, their analyses could correspond to the above formula even if they were not definite compounds but coprecipitated mixtures of nickel salts and solid polymers of isocyanides, because in most cases they were prepared by mixing the calculated amounts of reagents.

Nevertheless, the isolation of one unstable nickel (II) complex is reported[2]. When an acetone solution of and phenylisocyanide was strongly cooled for two days, diamagnetic brown crystals of a 1:1 adduct were isolated. Similar complexes were also obtained with tertiary phosphines, but not with acetonitrile or with benzonitrile. While it is reported that only π-accepting molecules can give adducts, the increase of the CN stretching frequency of the isocyanide in the complex *versus* the uncomplexed isocyanide is evidence for very small back-donation. By interaction of nickel (II) with donor molecules, the electron density on the metal atom is increased, while the actual positive charge on the four nitrogen atoms of the oxime is decreased. Correspondingly, the oxime C$=$N stretching frequency is lowered on going from the Ni^{II} complex to the 1:1 adduct, by up to 35 cm^{-1}. The isocyanide adduct can be dissolved in organic solvents, where it breaks down. As a solid it can be handled in the air only for a short time.

The lability of the nickel (II) adducts with isocyanides was brilliantly exploited to study the delocalization of the spin density into the π-orbitals of the ligand, when the latter was coordinated to nickel (II) acetylacetonate[3], by means of n.m.r.

It may be remarked here that the metals which form halogeno-carbonyls, such as $FeX_2(CO)_4$, $[PdCl_2(CO)]_2$ and $PtCl_2(CO)_2$, also form halogenoisocyanide compounds. These may or may not be of a type similar to the corresponding halogenocarbonyl, e.g. FeX_2-$(CNR)_4$, $PdX_2(CNR)_2$, $PtX_2(CNR)_2$ and $[Pt(CNR)_4][PtX_4]$, but are always very stable. The elements that, like nickel, chromium, molybdenum and tungsten, did not seem able to form carbonyl halides, had instead given very unstable and ill-defined isocyanide complexes in oxidation states other than zero. This consideration was made to explain the absence of stable salts of the cation $[Ni(CNR)_4]^{2+}$. However, the recent isolation of many carbonyl halides of Group VI elements means that the correlation may be unjustified.

Derivatives of nickel (I)

Derivatives of formally monovalent nickel are very interesting. By reaction of dicyclopentadienylnickel (II) and tetrakis(phenyl isocyanide)nickel (0) in boiling benzene, Pauson isolated[4] dimeric cyclopentadienylphenylisocyanidenickel (I). On the grounds of the infrared spectrum in dichloromethane (band at 2174 cm^{-1}), structure 1 was assigned to the compound.

$$
\begin{array}{ccc}
 & & R \\
 & & | \\
 & & N \\
 & & \| \\
H_5C_5 \diagdown \quad\quad CNR & & C \\
\quad\quad Ni{-}Ni \diagdown & C_5H_5Ni{-}{-}{-}{-}{-}{-}NiC_5H_5 \\
RNC \diagup \quad\quad C_5H_5 & & C \\
\quad\quad (1) & & \| \\
 & & N \\
 & & | \\
 & & R \\
 & & (2)
\end{array}
$$

More recently Pauson reformulated the compound as **2**, on the basis of a new recording of the infrared spectrum, this time in a KBr disc, since alteration took place in the chlorinated solvent[5].

Another formally monovalent nickel compound, $[C_5H_5Ni(CNC_6H_{11})]_2$, was prepared similarly, but at room temperature, by Yamamoto and Hagihara[6], while working on the polymerization of cyclohexyl isocyanide using various metallocenes as catalyst. The air-sensitive compound was also obtained from bis(cyclopentadienylcarbonylnickel) or from dicyclopentadienyl(acetylene)dinickel. The infrared spectral data in various solvents are available (see Table 8.1). From these data it was concluded that the isocyanide-bridged structure **2** is present in the solid state, like in the related carbonyl-bridged $[C_5H_5Ni(CO)]_2$, while in solution there is an equilibrium between structure **1** and **2**[6].

Derivatives of nickel (o)

The isocyanide derivatives of nickel (o) of formula $Ni(CNR)_4$ are among the most interesting isocyanide compounds because of their great stability and ease of formation.

It may be interesting to recall that they were the first products of complete substitution of a metal carbonyl to be obtained, since only partially substituted compounds were previously known. Afterwards it was found that many other ligands, all of the type with strong double-bonding character, are able to give completely substituted carbonyl-like compounds. A number of derivatives of trivalent phosphorous, namely PCl_3[7], PF_3[8], $PCl_2(C_6H_5)$[9], $PCl_2(OC_6H_5)$[9], PCl_2CH_3[10] form compounds of the type NiL_4, either by direct substitution from $Ni(CO)_4$ or in other ways. For instance dichloro-methylphosphine reacts with metallic nickel, analogously to carbon monoxide itself[10].

The tetrakis(aryl isocyanide)nickel compounds were obtained independently and almost at the same time (1947) by Hieber[11,12] and by Klages and Moenkemeyer[13,14,23], on reaction of aryl isocyanides with nickel carbonyl:

$$Ni(CO)_4 + 4\ CNR \rightarrow Ni(CNR)_4 + 4\ CO$$

The reaction takes place under mild conditions. It was found possible later[15] to prepare all the $Ni(CO)_{4-n}(CNPh)_n$ compounds ($n = 1, 2, 3, 4$). Although they were not always isolated in the pure state, the infrared spectra of the mixtures were such as to allow the assignment of the bands due to each component of the mixtures.

The infrared spectra of these mixed carbonyl isocyanide compounds were reported and studied by Bigorgne[15,16]. A subsequent paper by Horrocks[17] gave the force constants calculated on the infrared data of Bigorgne for all the reported $Ni(CO)_{4-n}(CNR)_n$ compounds ($n = 3, 2, 1$; $R = CH_3, C_2H_5, n\text{-}C_3H_7, C_6H_5$). The force constants were calculated on the assumption that the isonitrile group is an interacting ligand; the assumption was found to be strictly necessary in some of the reported cases.

Independently, the tetrakis(aryl isocyanide)nickel compounds were prepared by Malatesta and Sacco[18] from nickel (II) compounds and isocyanides. The first positive results were obtained by reacting the bis(dimethylglyoximato)nickel (II) with aryl isocyanides in the presence of hydrazine. The bis(dimethylglyoximato)nickel (II) was chosen as starting material because it was known that under a high pressure of carbon monoxide it disproportionates to nickel carbonyl and a dimethylglyoxime derivative of nickel (IV)[19]. An analogous disproportionation reaction was expected to take place in the presence of isocyanides; the addition of hydrazine had the purpose of reducing the Ni^{IV} as soon as it was formed. In fact, the reaction proceeded according to the equation:

$$2\ Ni(DMG)_2 + 8\ CNR + N_2H_4 \rightarrow 2\ Ni(CNR)_4 + 4(DMG)H + N_2$$

It was later seen that in the presence of hydrazine all nickel salts undergo an analogous reaction, provided the medium is alkaline, and that even the presence of hydrazine is not strictly necessary, since the tetra(aryl isocyanide)nickel compounds are also formed slowly from an alcoholic suspension of nickel hydroxide and an excess of aryl isocyanide. The reaction can be considered to be:

$$Ni(OH)_2 + 5\ CNR \rightarrow Ni(CNR)_4 + RNCO + H_2O$$

An alternative way was found recently[20]. Reaction of phenyl isocyanide with nickelocene in ether below 0°C gives $Ni(CNPh)_4$ in quantitative yields. The same author mentions that $K_4[Ni(CN)]_4$ reacts similarly.

The tetrakis(aryl isocyanide)nickel compounds are yellow crystalline substances, of moderate thermal stability, soluble in organic solvents. They are stable to air in the solid state, but decompose rapidly in solution. In the absence of air, however, the solutions are quite stable and the products can be recovered unaltered[14]. The tetrakis(aryl isocyanide)nickel compounds are hydrophobic and are not affected by aqueous solutions of strong mineral acids and bases. Even aqueous potassium cyanide and mixtures of potassium cyanide and hydroxylamine, which attack many other nickel complexes, are without effect on the tetrakis(aryl isocyanide)nickel compounds. On the other hand they are completely destroyed by fuming nitric acid and by bromine.

The exchange reaction between $^{14}CNPh$ and $Ni(CNPh)_4$ was studied[21]. It was found to be so fast that it was impossible to measure the rate, even at 4°C.

Unlike aryl isocyanides, alkyl isocyanides do not easily displace carbon monoxide from nickel tetracarbonyl. The reaction between $Ni(CO)_4$ and methyl isocyanide yielded a yellow crystalline product, which was formulated as the carbonyltris(methyl isocyanide)-nickel (o)[12]. The compound is remarkably stable. The residual molecule of carbon monoxide can be displaced slowly by a solution of iodine in pyridine, rapidly and quantitatively by heating with aryl isocyanides. The general properties of $Ni(CO)(CNCH_3)_3$ are similar to those of the tetraisocyanide compounds.

The infrared spectra of these idealized tetrahedral molecules (Table 8.1) show two strong infrared bands, while only one is required in a molecule of effective tetrahedral symmetry, i.e., the symmetry corresponding to a molecule without significant bending of each of the C—N—C groups. The values recorded for the CN stretching frequencies are much lower, by 80–150 cm^{-1}, than the value recorded for the free ligand, as required by a large amount of metal–carbon π-bonding[22].

Although derivatives of alkyl isocyanides are rather unstable in nonhydrocarbon solvents, it is possible to obtain mono-, di- and tetrasubstituted compounds starting from alkyl isocyanides and nickel carbonyl[16]. The monosubstituted compounds are sparingly soluble in saturated hydrocarbons, more soluble in ether and chloroform. $(CO)_2Ni(CNCH_3)_2$ is a white solid, sparingly soluble in the usual solvents.

PALLADIUM

Derivatives of palladium (ii)

Palladium halides react readily with aryliso cyanides, yielding stable and well-defined products which analyse as $PdX_2.2\ CNR$[24]. They are orange crystalline substances, with generally high melting points, soluble in methylene chloride, chloroform, benzene and nitrobenzene, very sparingly soluble in alcohol and in ether. They are diamagnetic, non-electrolytes, and monomeric in solution and must therefore be formulated as dihalogenobis(aryl isocyanide)-palladium (ii) compounds.

A square planar structure with dsp^2 orbitals may be attributed to these compounds. It cannot be said whether the crystalline products that were described have a *cis* or a *trans* configuration, but measurements of the dipole moments in benzene solution seem to indicate that in this solvent the *cis* form, or at least an equilibrium where the *cis* form prevails, is present[24].

The reported infrared data (see Table 8.3) are in agreement with the presence of the *cis* form in benzene and in chloroform solution, two CN bands being observed. All the other complexes showed only one CN band in the same solvents; therefore a *trans* structure was suggested for them.

No isocyanide derivatives of the palladium (ii) salts with non-coordinating anions could be prepared, which shows that neither the dicoordinated $[Pd(CNR)_2]^{2+}$ nor the tetracoordinated $[Pd(CNR)_4]^{2+}$ is stable. The instability of the latter may account for the fact that compounds $PdX_2(CNR)_2$, unlike the analogous Pt^{II} derivatives, exist only in the non-electrolyte monomeric form.

Derivatives of palladium (o)

The aryl isocyanide derivatives of palladium (o), of composition corresponding to $Pd(CNR)_2$, are the first known examples of isocyanide compounds of a zerovalent metal of which the corresponding pure carbonyl does not exist. They are also the only known case of formally coordinately unsaturated isocyanide compounds.

The preparation of these derivatives of palladium (o)[26,27,28,29,30] was possible only under strictly controlled conditions. In fact, the divalent derivatives, $PdX_2(CNR)_2$, cannot be reduced to the zerovalent state by strong reducing agents in acid, neutral or slightly alkaline medium. In strongly alkaline solution, the reduction takes place spontaneously, but only if two molecules of isocyanide per palladium atom are present. With slightly less than two moles of isocyanide, not even a trace of $Pd(CNR)_2$ is obtained, whereas a 5% excess over 2·5 moles results in a 50% yield.

As starting material for the preparation of the zerovalent compounds the diiodobis(aryl isocyanide)palladium compounds were chosen, because of their ease of preparation. The reaction sequence is presumed to be:

$$PdI_2(CNR)_2 + 2\ KOH \rightarrow Pd(OH)_2(CNR)_2 + 2\ KI$$

$$Pd(OH)_2(CNR)_2 + 3\ RNC \rightarrow Pd(CNR)_4 + RNCO + H_2O$$

$$Pd(CNR)_4 \rightarrow Pd(CNR)_2 + 2\ CNR$$

An alternative method of preparation makes use of cyclopentadienylcyclohexenylpalladium (II) or of cyclopentadienyl (π-allyl)-palladium (II). Addition of the ligand to the solution of the former in ether or of the latter in pentane precipitates $Pd(CNR)_2$[29,30].

The bis(aryl isocyanide)palladium (o) compounds prepared according to Malatesta's procedure are brown-black crystalline substances, stable to air, diamagnetic and practically insoluble in most solvents. The very few solvents which dissolve them, such as nitrobenzene or pyridine, cause complete decomposition, so that no molecular weight datum is available.

The same compounds prepared according to the other procedure, due to Fischer[29,30], are yellow and soluble in most organic solvents. Their infrared spectra show a weaker and a stronger CN band (reported in Table 8.3) plus a strong Pd—C and a medium Pd—N band at 516 and 436 respectively. This was taken as evidence for the isocyanide acting as a donor through the π-electron density of the CN bond, instead of through the carbon atom as is usual (see p. 29). The molecular weight of the compound was measured by cryoscopy in benzene and was found to be time-dependent, the minimum value found being that corresponding to a dimeric molecule. At room temperature and in the solid state the yellow compound changes into a dark one, with the same analyses. Two weeks are required for the CNPh complex but only a short time with the isopropyl isocyanide complex. These dark compounds were found to be insoluble in all the organic solvents tried, like Malatesta's compounds. On the other hand, Malatesta's compounds are soluble in pure, liquid aryl isocyanide, yielding yellow solutions. The compounds present in these solutions were not stable in the absence of excess isocyanide; they were not isolated.

The formation of the dark compounds as derivatives of palladium (o) was confirmed by their reaction with iodine. In alcoholic suspension they took up exactly one mole of iodine per mole of Pd-(CNR)$_2$, yielding PdI$_2$(CNR)$_2$, identical with the starting material used for the preparation of the zerovalent compounds, according to the reaction:

$$Pd(CNR)_2 + I_2 \rightarrow PdI_2(CNR)_2$$

On reaction with derivatives of trivalent phosphorous, such as triarylphosphines or triarylphosphites, a partial or complete displacement of the isocyanide occurred, and new mixed, symmetrical derivatives of zerovalent palladium were formed[31,32]. As shown by the following examples, the course of the reaction, as well as the products obtained, varied much with the substituting ligand:

$$(p\text{-}CH_3C_6H_4NC)_2Pd + 3\ (p\text{-}ClC_6H_4O)_3P \rightarrow$$
$$(p\text{-}CH_3C_6H_4NC)[(p\text{-}ClC_6H_4O)_3P]_3Pd + p\text{-}CH_3C_6H_4NC$$

$$(p\text{-}CH_3C_6H_4NC)_2Pd + 4\ (C_6H_4O)_3P \rightarrow [(C_6H_4O)_3P]_4Pd + 2\ p\text{-}CH_3C_6H_4NC$$

$$(p\text{-}CH_3C_6H_4NC)_2Pd + 3\ (p\text{-}ClC_6H_4)_3P \rightarrow$$
$$[(p\text{-}ClC_6H_4)_3P]_3Pd + 2\ p\text{-}CH_3C_6H_4NC$$

Among the hypotheses that have so far been advanced on the structure of the bis(isocyanide)palladium compounds, three are worth mentioning: (1) the palladium atom is coordinately unsaturated, forming only two linear bonds; polymerization to dark compounds then follows rapidly; (2) the palladium atom reaches the effective atomic number of xenon through four metallic bonds to other palladium atoms and two coordinate bonds to isocyanide molecules; (3) the isocyanide ligand is bridging. However, more work is required, especially an x-ray structure determination, to elucidate the structure of these compounds in a sure way.

PLATINUM

Compounds of the type PtX₂.2 CNR

The alkaline salts of the tetrahalogeno-, tetranitro- and tetracyano-platinic (II) acid react readily with isocyanides, yielding very stable compounds of general formula $PtX_2 . 2$ CNR (X = Cl, Br, I, NO_2, CN). Those in which X is Cl, Br, I and CN were obtained in two forms, one dimeric and ionic, $[Pt(CNR)_4][PtX_4]$, and the other monomeric and non-electrolyte, $PtX_2(CNR)_2$. The nitro derivative was obtained only in the non-ionic form. In several cases the monomeric $PtX_2(CNR)_2$ was isolated in two modifications of different colours and crystalline forms, possibly the *cis–trans* isomers expected for such compounds. The direct esterification of the acid $H_2[Pt(CN)_4]$ with ethanol was also tried, but the compounds obtained do not appear to be isocyanide derivatives[33].

Compounds with X = halogen

On treating a concentrated solution of sodium or potassium tetrachloroplatinate (II) or tetrabromoplatinate (II) or an alcoholic solution of sodium tetraiodoplatinate (II) with a slight excess of alkyl[34,35] or aryl isocyanides[36,37], intensely coloured substances separated at once. Their composition corresponded to $PtX_2(CNR)_2$. The alkyl derivatives are apparently isomorphous and practically insoluble in water; both are insoluble in practically all organic solvents. The chemical evidence suggests a saline structure, tetra-halogenoplatinates (II) of tetraisocyanideplatinum (II)[35]. In fact, an aqueous solution of the purple-red $PtCl_2(CNCH_3)_2$ or of the blue-violet $PtCl_2(CNC_6H_5)_2$ reacts with $[Pt(NH_3)_4]Cl_2$ yielding the green tetrachloroplatinate (II) of tetramminoplatinum (II) (Magnus' salt), thus proving the presence of the anion $[PtCl_4]^{2-}$. Although the chloride of tetraisocyanideplatinum was not isolated from the solution, the reaction may be considered to be:

$$[Pt(CNCH_3)_4][PtCl_4] + Pt(NH_3)_4Cl_2 \rightarrow [Pt(NH_3)_4][PtCl_4] + [Pt(CNCH_3)_4]Cl_2$$
  red, insoluble   green, insoluble

The presence of the cation $[Pt(CNR)_4]^{2+}$ was proved by addition of sodium picrate to the purple-red $PtCl_2(CNR)_2$ in aqueous solution; the picrate of tetrakis(methyl isocyanide)platinum (II) separated in yellow crystals sparingly soluble in water. The reaction may be written:

$$[Pt(CNCH_3)_4][PtCl_4] + 2\ NaOC_6H_2(NO_2)_3 \rightarrow$$
$$Na_2[PtCl_4] + [Pt(CNCH_3)_4][OC_6H_2(NO_2)_3]_2$$

On prolonged heating at 110–150°C in the dry state, or on boiling for several hours in chloroform, the red-violet salts, $[Pt(CNR)_4]$-$[PtX_4]$, are converted into pale yellow crystalline substances of identical composition[35,37]. These compounds are soluble in most organic solvents and insoluble in water. They are diamagnetic, non-electrolytes and monomeric in solution, and must be considered as the dihalogenodiisocyanideplatinum (II) compounds. Many of them were isolated in two crystal forms, often of slightly different colours, very easily converted into each other. It is not known whether they are just dimorphic forms or the *cis–trans* isomers expected for the square planar dihalogenodiisocyanideplatinum (II) compounds.

The yellow $PtCl_2(CNCH_3)_2$ gave the picrate of tetrakis(methyl-isocyanide)platinum (II) when an excess of methylisocyanide and then sodium picrate were added to the aqueous solution, according to the reactions:

$$PtCl_2(CNCH_3)_2 + 2\ CNCH_3 \rightarrow [Pt(CNCH_3)_4]Cl_2$$

$$[Pt(CNCH_3)_4]Cl_2 + 2\ NaOC_6H_2(NO_2)_3 \rightarrow$$
$$[Pt(CNCH_3)_4][OC_6H_2(NO_2)_3]_2 + 2\ NaCl$$

Compounds with X = NO₂

Potassium tetranitroplatinate (II) reacts with isocyanides in aqueous solution[37], yielding non-ionic, monomeric compounds of formula $Pt(NO_2)_2(CNR)_2$. These compounds exist in two forms of different colours and solubilities, easily converted into each other.

Compounds with X = CN

The reaction between potassium tetracyanoplatinate (II)[38] and methyl and ethyl isocyanide in water yields directly the monomeric dicyanodiisocyanideplatinum (II) compounds, $Pt(CN)_2(CNR)_2$.

They are fluorescent, colourless, crystalline substances, soluble in methanol, slightly soluble in water and chloroform. These compounds are extremely stable and are decomposed only by a concentrated solution of KCN. Unlike the analogous halogeno derivatives, they do not react with an excess of isocyanide to give the tetraisocyanideplatinum (II) cations. The methyl derivative was also obtained by alkylation of silver tetracyanoplatinate (II) with methyl iodide:

$$Ag_2[Pt(CN)_4] + CH_3I \rightarrow Pt(CN)_2(CNCH_3)_2 + 2\ AgI$$

The reaction between potassium tetracyanoplatinate (II) in aqueous solution and *tert*-butyl isocyanide gives as first product the tetracyanoplatinate (II) of tetrakis (*tert*-butyl isocyanide)platinum (II), in the form of bright red crystals, insoluble in all solvents. The salt-like structure of this compound was determined by treating it with sodium picrate in water; as in the case of the analogous chloro compounds, the picrate of tetrakis(*tert*-butyl isocyanide)platinum separated as yellow crystals. On long standing in water, alcohol or chloroform, the bright red salt, $[Pt(tert-C_4H_9NC)_4][Pt(CN)_4]$, was converted slowly into the non-ionic monomeric form, $Pt(CN)_2(tert-C_4H_9NC)_2$. The dicyanobis(*tert*-butyl isocyanide)platinum (II) is a colourless crystalline product, more soluble than its methyl or ethyl analogues. A mixture of the saline and the non-saline forms is obtained by treating platinum (II) cyanide with *tert*-butyl isocyanide.

The non-saline monomeric form is also formed, quite unexpectedly, in another way. The bright red crystalline tetrachloroplatinate of tetrakis(*tert*-butyl isocyanide)platinum, which can be easily prepared from aqueous $K_2[PtCl_4]$ and the isocyanide, behaves differently from the other compounds of this type. It does not change into the non-ionic yellow form on boiling in solvents, and on treating with an excess of isocyanides dissolves, giving the following reactions:

$$[PtL_4][PtCl_4] + L \rightarrow [PtL_4]Cl_2 \qquad (L = tert\text{-butylisocyanide})$$

$$[PtL_4]Cl_2 + H_2O \rightarrow Pt(CN)_2L_2 + 2\ C_4H_9OH + 2\ HCl$$

This is perhaps the only case of an isocyanide hydrolyzing neatly into hydrocyanic acid (or a simple derivative, i.e., coordinated CN^-) and an alcohol.

7 + I.C.M.

Compounds containing alkyl isocyanides and hydrazine

A remarkable series of complex salts of platinum (II) containing alkyl isocyanides and hydrazine was described by Chugaev and coworkers[39].

On treating a concentrated aqueous solution of sodium or potassium tetrachloroplatinate (II) first with methyl isocyanide and then with hydrazine, a bright red crystalline derivative was obtained, which was formulated as the chloride of di-μ-hydrazidobis(tetrakis-methyl isocyanide)platinum (II):

$$\left[\begin{array}{c} \text{NH—NH}_2 \\ (CH_3NC)_4Pt \qquad\qquad Pt(CNCH_3)_4 \\ \text{NH}_2\text{—NH} \end{array} \right] Cl_2$$

The corresponding iodide and perchlorate were obtained by treatment with sodium iodide or perchlorate. The iodide was obtained as a brown–red tetrahydrate, or as an emerald-green anhydrous salt; the perchlorate was obtained as a red dihydrate with green reflectances.

Analogous compounds were obtained with ethyl isocyanide. The chloride of di-μ-hydrazidobis(tetrakis-ethyl isocyanide)platinum (II) was not isolated, but the corresponding iodide, perchlorate, nitrate and tetrachloroplatinate (II) were obtained in a pure state. These compounds are all very stable; they form beautiful crystals, soluble in water, slightly soluble in alcohol. Their stability, as well as the conditions under which they are formed, is rather surprising. In fact, hydrazine in the presence of isocyanides would have been expected to reduce platinum (II) to the zerovalent isocyanide compounds, or—if these were not stable, at least to the metal.

Another peculiar feature of these compounds is the unusual coordination number—six—exhibited by platinum (II). In this respect it is interesting that on treatment with concentrated hydrochloric acid the salt $[Pt_2(N_2H_3)_2(CNCH_3)_8]Cl_2$ loses isocyanide giving the similar chloride of di-μ-hydrazidobis(tetrakis-methyl isocyanide)-platinum (II), $[Pt_2(N_2H_3)_2(CNCH_3)_4]Cl_2$, in which platinum (II) has the usual coordination number of four.

The salts of the cation $[Pt_2(N_2H_3)_2(CNCH_3)_4]^{2+}$ are stable yellow crystalline substances, less soluble in water than the corresponding salts of the cation $[Pt_2(N_2H_3)_2(CNCH_3)_8]^{2+}$. By action of alkali in the presence of methyl isocyanide, they are reconverted into the salts of di-μ-hydrazidobis(tetrakis-methyl isocyanide)-platinum (II), so that the reaction may be considered to be a sort of equilibrium:

$$[\text{Pt}_2(\text{N}_2\text{H}_3)_2(\text{CNCH}_3)_8]\text{Cl}_2 \underset{\text{OH}^- + \text{RNC}}{\overset{\text{HCl} (-\text{RNC})}{\rightleftarrows}} [\text{Pt}_2(\text{N}_2\text{H}_3)_2(\text{CNCH}_3)_4]\text{Cl}_2$$

red   yellow

On the whole, the structures attributed to these interesting compounds, though quite possible, do not seem thoroughly proved and deserve further investigation.

Table 8.1 Isocyanide compounds of nickel

Name	Formula	Colour and crystal form	M.p. °C	Infrared and other data	Ref.
(See text)	$C_8H_{12}B_2F_2N_4NiO_4$	Brown crystals	Unstable	2252(CN); spin-paired	2
Bis(cyclohexyl isocyanidecyclopentadienyl)nickel (t)	$[(CNC_6H_{11})(C_5H_5)Ni]_2$	Red-brown needles	155–156 (dec.)	Nujol:1870, 1830.n-C_6H_{14}:2140. C_6H_6:2140s, 1880w, 1840w	4, 5
Bis(phenyl isocyanidecyclopentadienyl)nickel (t)	$[(CNC_6H_5)(C_5H_5)Ni]_2$	—	91	KBr:1785, decomposed by CH_2Cl_2, CCl_4	6
Tricarbonylmethyl isocyanidenickel (o)	$Ni(CO)_3(CNCH_3)$	Colourless	—	$C_{16}H_{34}$:2187·5(CN); 2073·2(A), 2008·5(E), Raman, C_5H_{12}:2192, 2072, 2005	16, 17
Tricarbonylethyl isocyanidenickel (o)	$Ni(CO)_3(CNC_2H_5)$	—	—	$C_{16}H_{34}$:2178, 2017·5, 2007·8	16, 17
Tricarbonyl(n-butyl isocyanide)nickel (o)	$Ni(CO)_3(CNC_4H_9)$	—	—	$C_{16}H_{34}$:2174·3; 2071·3, 2007·0	16, 17
Tricarbonylphenyl isocyanidenickel (o)	$Ni(CO)_3(CNC_6H_5)$	Yellow	—	$C_{16}H_{34}$:2147; 2066; 2013 $CHCl_3$:2152; 2067, 2014 + 2004	15, 17
Dicarbonylbis(methyl isocyanide)nickel (o)	$Ni(CO)_2(CNCH_3)_2$	White	—	$C_{16}H_{34}$:2176·0(A), 2138·5(B)(CN); 2015·5(A), 1969·0(B)(CO)	16, 17
Dicarbonylbis(ethyl isocyanide)nickel (o)	$Ni(CO)_2(CNC_2H_5)_2$	White	—	$C_{16}H_{34}$:2116·5, 2131; 2013, 1968·0	15, 17

Name	Formula	Colour	M.p.	IR data	Refs.
Dicarbonylbis(n-butyl isocyanide)-nickel (o)	$Ni(CO)_2(CNC_4H_9)_2$	White	—	$C_{16}H_{34}$:2163·7, 2125·0; 2012, 1967·0	16, 17
Dicarbonylbis(phenyl isocyanide)-nickel (o)	$Ni(CO)_2(CNC_6H_5)_2$	—	—	$C_{16}H_{34}$:2142, 2085; 2015·5, 1984·5; $CHCl_3$:2146, 2095; 2018, 1976	16, 17
Carbonyltris(methyl isocyanide)-nickel (o)	$Ni(CO)(CNCH_3)_3$	Pale yellow crystals	110 dec.	$C_{16}H_3$:2165(A), 2104(E)(CN); 1952(A)(CO) Nujol:2183, 2128; 2016w, 1923	12, 16, 22
Carbonyltris(ethyl isocyanide)-nickel (o)	$Ni(CO)(CNC_2H_5)_3$	Pale yellow	—	$C_{16}H_{34}$:2155, 2096, 1950	16
Carbonyltris(n-butyl isocyanide)-nickel (o)	$Ni(CO)(CNC_4H_9)_3$	Pale yellow	—	$C_{16}H_{34}$:2153, 2090, 1950	16
Carbonyltris(phenyl isocyanide)-nickel (o)	$Ni(CO)(CNC_6H_5)_3$	—	—	$CHCl_3$:2142, 2070, 1971	15
Tetrakis(methyl isocyanide)-nickel (o)	$Ni(CNCH_3)_4$	Pale yellow crystals	—	—	16, 18
Tetrakis(phenyl isocyanide)-nickel (o)	$Ni(CNC_6H_5)_4$	Canary-yellow very long needles	202–204 dec.	$C_{16}H_{34}$:2136w(A_1), 2045, 2019, 1993(F_2) $CHCl_3$:2050, 1990 KBr:2029, 2013, 1998	12, 14, 15, 22
Tetrakis(p-tolyl isocyanide)-nickel (o)	$Ni(CNC_7H_7)_4$	Yellow needles	—	$CHCl_3$:2065, 2033	18, 22, 23
Tetrakis(p-chlorophenyl isocyanide)nickel (o)	$Ni(CNC_6H_4Cl)_4$	—	—	$CHCl_3$:2049, 2008	22
Tetrakis(2-naphthyl isocyanide)-nickel (o)	$Ni(CNC_{10}H_7)_4$	Yellow-red needles	—	—	23
Tetrakis(p-ethoxyphenyl isocyanide)nickel (o)	$Ni(CNC_8H_9O)_4$	Pale-yellow fine needles	206–208 dec.	—	23

Table 8.2   Isocyanide compounds of palladium

Name	Formula	Colour and crystals form	M.p. or dec. temp. °C	Ref.
Bis(phenyl isocyanide)palladium (o)	$Pd(CNC_6H_5)_2$	Dark brown leaflets	170–190 (dec.)	27
	$Pd(CNC_6H_5)_2$	Yellow needles	107–110 (dec.)	29, 30
	$Pd(CNC_6H_5)_2$	Red powder	—	40
Bis(isopropyl isocyanide)palladium (o)	$Pd(CNC_3H_7)_2$	Yellow-brown	55–56 (dec.)	29, 30
Bis(p-tolyl isocyanide)palladium (o)	$Pd(CNC_7H_7)_2$	Dark brown leaflets	150–160 (dec.)	27
Bis(p-anisyl isocyanide)palladium (o)	$Pd(CNC_7H_7O)_2$	Dark brown leaflets	160–170 (dec.)	27
p-Tolyl isocyanidetris[tris(p-chlorophenylphosphite)]palladium (o)	$Pd(CNC_7H_7)[P(OC_6H_4Cl)_3]_3$	White needles	105	27
p-Anisyl isocyanidetris[tris(p-chlorophenylphosphine)]palladium (o)	$Pd(CNC_7H_7O)[P(C_6H_4Cl)_3]_3$	Colourless crystals	90–100	32
p-Anisyl isocyanidetris(triphenylphosphite)palladium (o)	$Pd(CNC_7H_7O)[P(OC_6H_5)_3]_3$	Colourless crystals	105–110	32
p-Anisyl isocyanidetris[tris(p-chlorophenylphosphite)]palladium (o)	$Pd(CNC_7H_7O)[P(OC_6H_3Cl)_3]_3$	Colourless crystals	100–105	32
Diiodobis(p-anisyl isocyanide)palladium (II)	$PdI_2(CNC_7H_7O)_2$	Orange needles	—	24
Dichlorobis(p-tolyl isocyanide)palladium (II)	$PdCl_2(CNC_7H_7)_2$	Pale yellow needles	—	24
Dibromobis(p-tolyl isocyanide)palladium (II)	$PdBr_2(CNC_7H_7)_2$	Pale yellow needles	—	24
Diiodobis(p-tolyl isocyanide)palladium (II)	$PdI_2(CNC_7H_7)_2$	Orange needles	—	24
Diiodobis(p-anisyl isocyanide)palladium (II)	$PdI_2(CNC_7H_7O)_2$	Orange needles	—	24
Diiodobis(p-chlorophenyl isocyanide)palladium (II)	$PdI_2(CNC_6H_4Cl)_2$	Orange needles	—	24

Table 8.3 Infrared CN stretching frequencies for isocyanide complexes of palladium

Compound	ν(CN) nujol	ν(CN) CHCl$_3$	ν(CN) benzene	Ref.
cis-Pd(CNPh)$_2$Cl$_2$	$\begin{cases}2237\\2222\end{cases}$	2230 2218	insol.	25
trans-Pd(CNPh)$_2$Br$_2$	2200	2200	2200	25
trans-Pd(CNPh)$_2$I$_2$	2192	2192	2190	25
trans-Pd(p-CH$_3$C$_6$H$_4$CN)$_2$Cl$_2$	2210	2208	insol.	25
trans-(p-CH$_3$C$_6$H$_4$CN)$_2$PdBr$_2$	2208	2205	2205	25
trans-(p-CH$_3$C$_6$H$_4$CN)$_2$PdI$_2$	2200	2195	2197	25
black Pd(CNPh)$_2$	2099	insol.	insol.	25
yellow Pd(CNPh)$_2$	$\begin{cases}2125\text{vw}\\1957\text{vs}\end{cases}$	—	—	29

All bands are strong, unless stated otherwise.

Table 8.4   Isocyanide compounds of platinum

Name	Formula	Colour and crystal form	M.p. or dec. temp. °C	Ref.
Dichlorobis(methyl isocyanide)platinum (II)	$PtCl_2(CNCH_3)_2$	Colourless crystals	233 (dec.)	35
Dicyanobis(methyl isocyanide)platinum (II)	$Pt(CN)_2(CNCH_3)_2$	Colourless needles		38
Dicyanobis(ethyl isocyanide)platinum (II)	$Pt(CN)_2(CNC_2H_5)_2$	Colourless needles		38
Dicyanobis(tert-butyl isocyanide)platinum (II)	$Pt(CN)_2(CNC_4H_9)_2$	Yellow crystals		38
Dichlorobis(ethyl isocyanide)platinum (II)	$PtCl_2(CNC_2H_5)_2$	Colourless crystals Yellow needles	257–258 219–220	37 41
Dibromobis(phenyl isocyanide)platinum (II)	$PtBr_2(CNC_6H_5)_2$	Colourless crystals	245	37
Diiodobis(phenyl isocyanide)platinum (II)	$PtI_2(CNC_6H_5)_2$	Yellow large crystals Yellow fine needles	241	37
Bis(triiodo)bis(phenyl isocyanide)platinum (II)	$Pt(I_3)_2(CNC_6H_5)_2$	Purple-red needles		37
Dinitrobis(phenyl isocyanide)platinum (II)	$Pt(NO_2)_2(CNC_6H_5)_2$	Yellow needles Dark red needles	155 (dec.)	37
Tetrakis(methyl isocyanide)platinum (II) tetrachloroplatinate (II)	$[Pt(CNCH_3)_4][PtCl_4]$	Red tablets		35
Tetrakis(methyl isocyanide)platinum (II) picrate	$[Pt(CNCH_3)_4][OC_6H_2(NO_2)_3]_2$	Yellow crystals		35
Tetrakis(tert-butyl isocyanide)platinum (II) picrate	$[Pt(CNC_4H_9)_4][OC_6H_2(NO_2)_3]_2$	Yellow crystals		35
Tetrakis(tert-butyl isocyanide)platinum (II) tetrachloroplatinate (II)	$[Pt(CNC_4H_9)_4][PtCl_4]$	Red crystals		35

Tetrakis(phenyl isocyanide)platinum (II) tetrachloroplatinate	$[Pt(CNC_6H_5)_4][PtCl_4]$	Blue-violet powder	36, 37
Tetrakis(phenyl isocyanide)platinum (II) tetrabromoplatinate	$[Pt(CNC_6H_5)_4][PtBr_4]$	Brown-violet powder	37
Di-μ-hydrazidobis[bis(methyl isocyanide)-platinum (II)] chloride with 2 moles HCl	$[(CH_3NC)_2Pt(NHNH_2)_2Pt(CNCH_3)_2]Cl_2 . 2\ HCl$	Colourless prisms	39
Di-μ-hydrazidobis[bis(ethyl isocyanide)-platinum (II)] chloride with 2 moles HCl	$[(C_2H_5NC)_2Pt(NHNH_2)_2Pt(CNC_2H_5)_2]Cl_2 . 2\ HCl$	White needles	39
Di-μ-hydrazidobis[tetrakis-(methyl isocyanide)platinum (II)] chloride octahydrate	$[(CH_3NC)_4Pt(NHNH_2)_2Pt(CNCH_3)_4]Cl_2 . 8\ H_2O$	Red prisms	39
Di-μ-hydrazidobis[tetrakis(methyl isocyanide)platinum (II)] iodide tetrahydrate	$[(CH_3NC)_4Pt(NHNH_2)_2Pt(CNCH_3)_4]I_2 . 4\ H_2O$	Brown-red needles	39
Di-μ-hydrazidobis[tetrakis(methyl isocyanide)platinum (II)] perchlorate dihydrate	$[(CH_3NC)_4Pt(NHNH_2)_2Pt(CNCH_3)_4](ClO_4)_2 . 2\ H_2O$	Red needles	39
Di-μ-hydrazidobis[tetrakis(ethyl isocyanide)platinum (II)] chloride	$[(C_2H_5NC)_4Pt(NHNH_2)_2Pt(CNC_2H_5)_4]Cl_2$	Yellow-orange needles	39
Di-μ-hydrazidobis[tetrakis(ethyl isocyanide)platinum (II)] iodide	$[(C_2H_5NC)_4Pt(NHNH_2)_2Pt(CNC_2H_5)_4]I_2$	Yellow needles	39
Di-μ-hydrazidobis[tetrakis(ethyl isocyanide)-platinum (II)] nitrate dihydrate	$[(C_2H_5NC)_4Pt(NHNH_2)_2Pt(CNC_2H_5)_4](NO_3)_2 . 2\ H_2O$	Red prisms	39
Di-μ-hydrazidobis[tetrakis(ethyl isocyanide)-platinum (II)] perchlorate	$[(C_2H_5NC)_4Pt(NHNH_2)_2Pt(CNC_2H_5)_4](ClO_4)_2$	Red prisms and needles	39
Di-μ-hydrazidobis[tetrakis(ethyl isocyanide)-platinum (II)] tetrachloroplatinate (II)	$[(C_2H_5NC)_4Pt(NHNH_2)_2Pt(CNC_2H_5)_4][PtCl_4]$	Red crystals	39

7*

REFERENCES

1. L. Malatesta, *Gazz. Chim. Ital.*, **77**, 340 (1947).
2. G. N. Schrauzer, *Chem. Ber.*, **95**, 1438 (1962).
3. W. D. Horrocks, Jr., R. C. Taylor and G. N. La Mar, *J. Am. Chem. Soc.*, **86**, 303 (1964).
4. P. L. Pauson and W. H. Stubbs, *Angew. Chem.*, **74**, 466 (1962); *Angew. Chem. (Int. Edit.)*, **1**, 333 (1962).
5. K. K. Joshi, O. S. Mills, P. L. Pauson, B. W. Shaw and W. H. Stubbs, *Chem. Comm.*, **1965**, 181.
6. Y. Yamamoto and N. Hagihara, *Bull. Chem. Soc. Japan*, **39**, 1084 (1966).
7. J. W. Irvine and G. Wilkinson, *Science*, **113**, 742 (1951).
8. G. Wilkinson, *J. Am. Chem. Soc.*, **73**, 5501 (1951).
9. L. Malatesta and A. Sacco, *Ann. Chim. (Italy)*, **44**, 134 (1954).
10. L. D. Quin, *J. Am. Chem. Soc.*, **79**, 3681 (1957).
11. W. Hieber, *Z. Naturforsch.*, **5b**, 129 (1950).
12. W. Hieber and E. Boeckly, *Z. anorg. Chem.*, **262**, 344 (1950).
13. F. Klages and K. Moenkemeyer, *Naturwissenschaften*, **37**, 210 (1950).
14. F. Klages and K. Moenkemeyer, *Chem. Ber.*, **83**, 501 (1950).
15. M. Bigorgne and L. Rassat, *Bull. Soc. Chim. France*, **1963**, 295.
16. M. Bigorgne and A. Bouquet, *J. Organomet. Chem.*, **1**, 101 (1963).
17. G. R. Van Hecke and W. D. Horrocks, Jr., *Inorg. Chem.*, **5**, 1960 (1966).
18. L. Malatesta and A. Sacco, *Atti Accad. naz. Lincei, Rend. Classe Sci. fis. mat. nat.*, [*VIII*], **11**, 379 (1951).
19. W. Hieber and R. Brueck, *Z. anorg. Chem.*, **269**, 28 (1952).
20. H. Behrens and K. Meyer, *Z. Naturforsch.*, **21b**, 489 (1966).
21. G. Cetini and O. Gambino, *Ann. Chim. (Italy)*, **53**, 236 (1963).
22. F. A. Cotton and F. Zingales, *J. Am. Chem. Soc.*, **83**, 351 (1961).
23. F. Klages, K. Moenkemeyer and R. Heinle, *Chem. Ber.*, **85**, 109 (1952).
24. M. Angoletta, *Ann. Chim. (Italy)*, **45**, 970 (1955).
25. F. Canziani, F. Cariati and U. Sartorelli, *Ist. Lombardo (Rend. Sc.)*, **A98**, 564 (1964).
26. L. Malatesta, *Atti Accad. naz. Lincei, Rend. Classe Sci. fis. mat. nat.*, [*VIII*], **16**, 364 (1954).
27. L. Malatesta, *J. Chem. Soc.*, **1955**, 3924.
28. L. Malatesta, *Rec. Trav. Chim.*, **75**, 644 (1956).
29. E. O. Fischer and H. Werner, *Chem. Ber.*, **95**, 703 (1962).
30. *German Patent* 1,181,708; *Chem. Abstr.*, **62**, 4947c (1965).
31. L. Malatesta and M. Angoletta, *Atti Accad. naz. Lincei, Rend. Classe Sci. fis. mat. nat.*, [*VIII*], **19**, 44 (1955).
32. L. Malatesta and M. Angoletta, *J. Chem. Soc.*, **1957**, 1186.
33. M. Freund, *Chem. Ber.*, **21**, 937 (1888).
34. L. Chugaev, *Compt. Rend.*, **159**, 188 (1914).
35. L. Chugaev and P. Teearu, *Chem. Ber.*, **47**, 568 (1914).
36. K. A. Hofmann and G. Bugge, *Chem. Ber.*, **40**, 1772 (1907).
37. L. Ramberg, *Chem. Ber.*, **40**, 2578 (1907).
38. L. Chugaev and P. Teearu, *Chem. Ber.*, **47**, 2643 (1914).

39. L. Chugaev, M. Skanavy Grigorieva and A. Posniak, *Z. anorg. Chem.*, **148**, 37 (1925).
40. L. Malatesta, unpublished results.
41. K. A. Jensen, *Z. anorg. Chem.*, **231**, 365 (1937)

APPENDIX

ADDITION TO CHAPTER 1

New data are available about the stability of isocyanides, both toward hydrolysis[1], rearrangement to cyanide[2,3] and polymerization.

The cationic polymerization of t-butyl, cyclohexyl, phenyl and 2-naphthyl isocyanide was investigated; the pale yellow polymer was found to be a poly-Schiff base, soluble in chloroform and tetrahydrofuran, molecular weight 4,000. Acid hydrolysis of the polymer afforded amine hydrochloride. t-Butyl and cyclohexyl isocyanide were not polymerized by $BF_3 . Et_2O$[4]. However, cyclohexylisocyanide is reported by a different source to yield high-melting solids on polymerization initiated by $BF_3 . Et_2O$; no copolymer, but only mixtures of homopolymers were obtained when other monomers were present in the reaction mixture[5]. Only diazomethane at $-78°$ afforded a copolymer[6]. Anionic polymerization is very slow. Attempts at polymerization initiated by azabisisobutyronitrile gave very low yields of $Me_2C(CN)(C=NPh)_3C(CN)Me_2$. Metal carbonyl, metallocenes and cyclopentadienyl metal carbonyl were successful polymerization catalysts for phenyl isocyanide: nickel tetracarbonyl and dicobalt octacarbonyl were highly active, iron pentacarbonyl weakly active, while group VI and dimanganese decacarbonyl were inactive. t-Butyl isocyanide was not polymerized by simple metal carbonyl, but only by the other compounds listed[4].

If the typical smell were not sufficient, microgram quantities of isocyanides can be detected qualitatively on a filter paper by using a colorimetric test[7].

Additional data are available on ^{14}N nuclear magnetic resonance (cf. Table 1.7 (p. 18) and ref. 81, Chapter 1). McFarlane[8] determined the reduced coupling constant between nitrogen and carbon connected by a single bond in methyl isocyanide; he found that it is positive, in agreement with theory. The signs of geminal and vicinal couplings between hydrogen and nitrogen are negative and positive, respectively. Witanowsky[9] compared the ^{14}N chemical shifts of nitriles, isocyanides and cyanide ion; he found that the relative chemical shifts between the resonances can be accounted for theoretically.

There is now a paper devoted to the electron spin resonance spectra of anions derived from p- and m-phenylene diisocyanide, 4,4′-biphenyl diisocyanide, 1,5-naphthalene diisocyanide and isocyanobenzonitrile[10] in addition to the data already available on the anion derived from 2,6-di-t-butyl-4-isocyanophenol[11].

Generalized mean square amplitudes of vibration, shrinkage effects and Coriolis coupling constants for methyl isocyanide are now available[12]. The microwave spectrum of ethyl isocyanide is the subject of a dissertation[13].

ADDITION TO CHAPTER 2

The infrared criterion (p. 26) was used to derive a classification of π-donor strength of metals in monosubstituted metal carbonyls. A comparison was made between the wave numbers of a ligand in monosubstituted metal carbonyl and the wave number of the same ligand before coordination[14]. The ligand employed included phenyl and cyclohexyl isocyanides; the results were found equally valid for dimethylsulphoxide and tetramethylenesulphide. The donor ability was found to fall in the order:

$$Fe(CO)_4 < Mo(CO)_5 \cong W(CO)_5 \cong Cr(CO)_5$$
$$< (dimethyltherephthalate)Cr(CO)_5 \cong C_5H_5Mn(CO)_2 < C_6H_6Cr(CO)_2$$
$$< (mesitylene)Cr(CO)_2 < (hexamethylbenzene)Cr(CO)_2$$

ADDITION TO CHAPTER 3

During investigations on the catalytic properties of copper compounds, a novel dimerization of α,β-unsaturated carbonyl compounds was discovered in the presence of isocyanide[15]:

$$R'-CH=CH-COR'' \xrightarrow[\text{3 hours}]{90°} \begin{array}{c} R'-CH=C-COR'' \\ | \\ R'-CH-CH_2COR'' \end{array}$$

The dimerization of crotonitrile, but not of acrylates, methacrylates and cinnamates, was equally successful in the presence of cuprous oxide and cyclohexyl isocyanide; neither of these two latter compounds alone is an effective catalyst.

It was also found by the same group of Japanese workers that it was not only amines, alcohols and thiols which react with isocyanides in the presence of copper catalyst[16,17]. With this catalyst it was found possible to insert the carbon atom of an isocyanide between the silicon and hydrogen of a silane compound, e.g.:

$$C_6H_{11}NC + (CH_3)_3SiH \xrightarrow[5\,h]{100°} (CH_3)_3SiCH{=}NC_6H_{11}$$

The reaction was carried out under nitrogen and in a benzene solution in which copper(II) acetylacetonate was present. Hexachloroplatinic acid, which is known to be an efficient catalyst for hydrosilation of olefins, was not a catalyst for the insertion.

The reaction between anhydrous tin(IV) or silicon(IV) chloride and p-tolyl isocyanide in toluene solution afforded a polymeric material[18].

ADDITION TO CHAPTERS 4 AND 5

Following the discovery of carbene complexes, the reaction of (methylmethoxycarbene)pentacarbonylchromium(0) with cyclohexyl and methyl isocyanide was investigated. The yellow 1:1 'adduct' was shown to have an aziridine structure, on the basis of spectral and chemical evidence[19]:

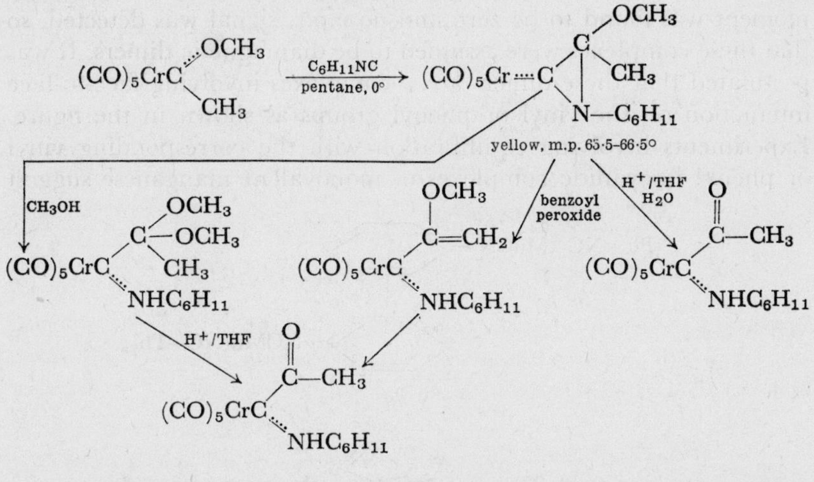

The derivatives of groups VI metal carbonyls with hydrocyanic and isohydrocyanic acid were fully investigated by Guttenberger[20] (cf. ref. 10, Chapter 1). His results can be summarized as follows:

$$M(CO)_6 \xrightarrow{THF} M(CO)_5THF \xrightarrow{HCN} (CO)_5M(NCH)$$

$$\Big\downarrow \text{piperidine}$$

$$(CO)_5M(CNH) \xleftarrow[CH_2Cl_2]{HCl} [(CO)_5MCN]^-$$

The properties of the above complexes are in agreement with those reported independently by King[21] (cf. Tables 4.1, 4.2, 4.4 and 4.5).

Similar compounds have been prepared in the case of manganese, and similar investigations have been announced on the protonation of $[C_5H_5V(CO)_3CN]^-$ and $[C_6H_6Cr(CO)_2CN]^{-}$ [22]:

$$C_5H_5Mn(CO)_3 \xrightarrow[\text{methanol}]{CN^-, 30°} [C_5H_5Mn(CO)_2CN]^-$$

	$C_5H_5Mn(CO)_2(CNH)$	$C_5H_5Mn(CO)_2(CND)$
m.p.	76	77
ν(CN)	2016 vs	1968 vs
ν(NH) or (ND)	3413m	2618m
ν(CO)	1819 and 1859 vs	1819 and 1859 vs
τ(C$_5$H$_5$)	5·83	5·92
τ(NH)	5·18 broad	—

(with H_3PO_4 yielding $C_5H_5Mn(CO)_2(CNH)$ and D_3PO_4 yielding $C_5H_5Mn(CO)_2(CND)$)

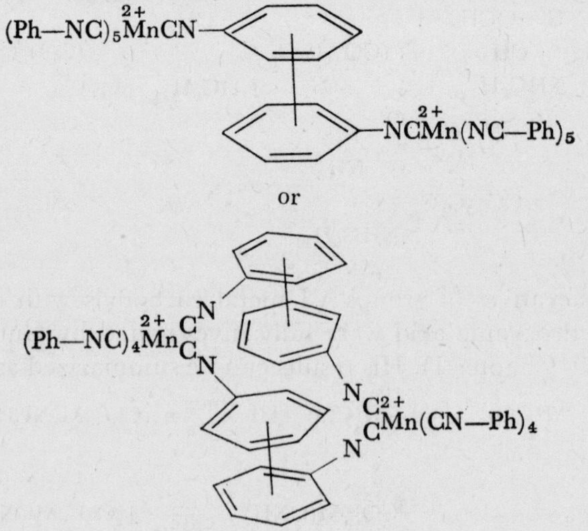

The magnetic behaviour of $[MnL_6]^{2+}$ derivatives was found to be normal (1·95–2·1 BM in acetonitrile solution at room temperature) for the complexes where L is a saturated aliphatic isocyanide. Surprisingly, when L was a phenyl or allyl isocyanide, the magnetic moment was found to be zero and no e.p.r. signal was detected, so that these complexes were assumed to be diamagnetic dimers. It was postulated that these dimers are π-complexes involving face-to-face interaction on the vinyl or phenyl groups as shown in the figure. Experiments involving equilibration with the corresponding vinyl or phenyl isocyanide complexes of monovalent manganese suggest that a paramagnetic dimer is involved in this case. The stability of the dimeric complexes was explained as being due to electron exchange and spin pairing[23].

Mass spectral data are now available for $C_5H_5Mn(CO)_2$-(CNC_6H_{11})[24] and for $W(CO)_5(CNC_6H_5)$[25]. While the primary fragmentation of the related $C_5H_5Mn(CO)_3^+$ results in a stepwise loss of carbonyl ligands, the first decomposition step of the mono-substituted derivatives is a simultaneous splitting of both carbonyl groups. Besides, both fragments of the isocyanide ligands, that is cyclohexene and isohydrocyanic acid, can be found on the cyclo-pentadienylmanganese moiety, as $C_5H_5MnC_6H_{10}^+$ or as C_5H_5Mn-$(CNH)^+$. A close relationship was found between the ionization energies and the carbonyl stretching frequencies of the C_5H_5Mn-$(CO)_2L$ compounds as well as the ionization-potential values of the uncoordinated ligands and the corresponding complexes.

ADDITION TO CHAPTERS 6 AND 7

The preparation of the assumed square planar $[FeL_4](ClO_4)_2$ compounds (p. 107) could not be repeated when L = p-tolyliso-cyanide; the reaction product was found to be $[FeL_5](ClO_4)_2$. Attempts to obtain the tetracoordinated compound by reaction of FeL_4Cl_2 (either isomer) with excess sodium perchlorate yielded $[FeL_4Cl](ClO_4)$: both compounds are believed to be examples of five coordinate and diamagnetic Fe (II) complexes. The 1:1 adduct between FeL_4Cl_2 and $HgCl_2$ (p. 106) was also reinvestigated, to-gether with additional new 1:1 adducts formed with $CdCl_2$ or $SnCl_4$. An ionic structure, $[FeL_4(solvent)_2]HgCl_4$, is likely to be present in donor solvents, while chloride bridges are present in the solid state and in solution of non-donor solvents[18].

Other five-coordinate complexes of cobalt (II) were obtained: $[CoL_4P]^+$ and $[CoL_3P_2]^{2+}$, where L is p-tolylisocyanide and P is a tertiary phosphine. These complexes are likely to have trigonal bipyramidal structure, with the phosphorous atom on the threefold axis of rotation, on the basis of infrared and n.m.r. data[26].

ADDITION TO CHAPTER 8

Recent results by Japanese workers[27] add zerovalent nickel and palladium complexes to the list of molecules able to react with molecular oxygen yielding 'adducts' of the type of Vaska's O_2Ir-$(CO)Cl(PPh_3)_2$. They reported the synthesis of pale green NiL_2O_2, from ethereal NiL_4 and oxygen at $-20°$. The solid complex ($\nu(CN)$: 2180; $\nu(O—O)$ 898 cm^{-1}) decomposes slowly at room temperature, rapidly at 95°, and immediately in benzene or chloroform solution. On the basis of infrared evidence, including labelling with $^{18}O_2$, the two oxygen atoms coordinate to the metal as a peroxo group, as in Vaska's compound[28]. A similar complex with rhodium, RhO_2Cl-$(t\text{-BuNC})(PPh_3)_2$ is mentioned by the same workers[27]. Both the rhodium and the nickel complex are active catalysts in the oxidation of isocyanide to isocyanate, and the reaction may be formulated as follows:

$$Ni(t\text{-BuNC})_4 \xrightarrow{O_2} \underset{(t\text{-BuNC})}{\overset{(t\text{-BuNC})}{Ni}} \overset{O}{\underset{O}{\diagup\diagdown}} \xrightarrow{t\text{-BuNC}} t\text{-BuNCO} + Ni(t\text{-BuNC})_4$$

The first reported complex containing both isocyanide and hydride ligand was obtained by Mays[29] by reaction of t-BuNC with $trans$-$PtHCl(PEt_3)_2$. The complex, $[trans\text{-}PtH(CNBu)(PEt_3)_2](ClO_4)$ has $\nu(CN)$ at 2203 and no evident ν (PtH); the evidence for the hydride is given by an n.m.r. signal at 17.09 τ in chloroform solution.

Infrared data are available for one of the $cis\text{-}PtL_2Cl_2$ compounds, obtained in the usual way; the yellow crystals, m.p. 195–197°, have absorption maxima at 2239 and 2208 (ν_{CN}), and 349 and 329 (ν_{Pt-Cl}) in chloroform solution, at 338 and 317 in nujol mull[30].

REFERENCES

1. M. Khalifa, *J. Pharm. Sci. U. Arab Rep.*, **6**, 133 (1965); *Chem. Abstr.*, **68**, 12069 (1968).
2. G. V. Van Dine and R. Hoffmann, *J. Am. Chem. Soc.*, **90**, 3227 (1968).
3. D. C. Taddy and B. S. Rabinovitch, *J. Chem. Phys.*, **48**, 1282 (1968).
4. Y. Yamamoto, T. Takizawa and N. Hagihara, *Nippon Kagaku Zasshi*, **87**, 1355 (1966); *Chem. Abstr.*, **67**, 32997 (1967).
5. R. W. Stackmann, *J. Macromol. Sci.*, part A, **2**, 225 (1968).
6. S. Iwatsuki, K. Ito and Y. Yamashita, *Kogyo Kagaku Zasshi*, **70**, 1822 (1967); *Chem. Abstr.*, **68**, 10558 (1968).
7. E. V. Crabtree, E. J. Poziomek and D. J. Hoy, *Talanta*, **14**, 857 (1967).
8. W. McFarlane, *J. Chem. Soc.*, part A, **1967**, 1660.
9. M. Witanowsky, *Tetrahedron*, **23**, 4299 (1967).
10. G. F. Longster, J. Myatt and P. F. Todd, *J. Chem. Soc.*, part B, **1967**, 612.
11. A. Rieker, K. Schleffer, R. Mayer, B. Narr and E. Mueller, *Ann. Chem.*, **693**, 10 (1966).

12. K. Venkateswarlu, K. V. Rajalakshmi and C. Puroshotamam, *Bull. Soc. Roy. Sci. Liege*, **36**, 583 (1967).
13. R. J. Anderson, *Dissertation Abstr.*, **B28**, 858 (1967); *Chem. Abstr.*, **68**, 44568 (1968).
14. W. Strohmeier, J. F. Guttenberger and F. J. Mueller, *Z. Naturforsch.*, **22b**, 1091 (1967).
15. T. Saegusa, Y. Ito, S. Kobayashi and K. Hirota, *J. Am. Chem. Soc.*, **89**, 2240 (1967).
16. T. Saegusa, Y. Ito, S. Kobayashi, K. Hirota and T. Shimizu, *J. Org. Chem.*, **88**, 544 (1968).
17. T. Saegusa, Y. Ito, S. Kobayashi and S. Tomita, *Chem. Comm.*, **1968**, 273.
18. Unpublished data.
19. R. Aumann and E. O. Fischer, *Chem. Ber.*, **101**, 954 (1968).
20. J. F. Guttenberger, *Chem. Ber.*, **101**, 403 (1968).
21. R. B. King, *Inorg. Chem.*, **6**, 25 (1967).
22. E. O. Fischer and R. J. J. Schneider, *J. Organomet. Chem.*, **12**, P27 (1968).
23. D. S. Matteson and R. A. Bailey, *J. Am. Chem. Soc.*, **89**, 6389 (1967).
24. J. Mueller and M. Herberhold, *J. Organomet. Chem.*, **13**, 399 (1968).
25. S. Pignataro, A. Foffani, G. Innorta and G. Di Stefano, *Commun. Intern. Mass Spectrometry Conf.*, Berlin, 1967; *J. Organomet. Chem.*, **14**, 165 (1968).
26. M. Rossi, private communication.
27. S. Otsuka, A. Nakamura and Y. Tatsuno, *Chem. Comm.*, **1967**, 836.
28. K. Hirota, M. Yamamoto, S. Otsuka, A. Nakamura and Y. Tatsuno, *Chem. Comm.*, **1968**, 533.
29. M. J. Church and M. J. Mays, *Chem. Comm.*, **1968**, 435.
30. M. Baird, private communication.

AUTHOR INDEX

This author index is designed to enable the reader to locate the author's name and work with the aid of the reference numbers appearing in the text. The page numbers are printed in normal type in ascending numerical order, followed by numbers in italics referring to the pages on which the references are actually listed. The numbers in brackets are the reference numbers.

189

SUBJECT INDEX

Acetylene, displacement by isocyanide 161

Acetylenic derivatives 45

Addition reactions of isocyanides and of hydrocyanic acid, in the presence of copper compounds 4, 38, 40, 42

Adducts of metal halides with RNC complexes 106–107, 135, 141

Alcohols
from isocyanide complexes 169
reactions with $H_3Co(CN)_6$ 133
reaction with $H_2Pt(CN)_4$ 167
unsaturated, reactions with RNC 42

Alkylation
of cyanocomplexes 42, 46–48, 60, 66, 67, 69, 73, 74, 75, 97–104, 107, 114, 132, 169
of organometallic cyanocompounds 24, 64, 69, 75

Aluminum alkyls
adducts with RNC 52
reaction with isocyanide complexes 61

Ammonia, displacement by isocyanide 24, 45, 64

Aromatic ligands in complexes
preparation of the complexes 65–66
spectra 79

Benzyl isocyanide, preparation 11

Bond refraction 9

π-Bonding 25, 27, 64, 65, 66, 70–72, 88, 112, 143, 163
spectrochemical series 24–25, 65–66, 70–72, 88

Boron hydrides
reaction with isocyanides 52

Boron hydrides—*cont.*
reaction with rhenium isocyanide complexes 90
reaction with iron isocyanide complexes 108

Bridging isocyanide groups 28, 108, 161

t-Butyl isocyanide, preparation 10

Cadmium halides, adducts with cobalt isocyanide complexes 135

Carbylamine reaction 4

Carbodiimides 110

Carbon monoxide
displacement by isocyanides 23, 24, 62, 68, 69, 88, 90, 107, 109, 111, 112, 114, 142, 144, 146, 161, 162
displacement by $R_3M(NC)$ compounds 109–110
effect of the solvent in the displacement of 88
not displaced by isocyanides 50, 163

Catalysis by isocyanide complexes 28, 42, 61, 69, 75

Chloride bridged complexes
of gold (III) 44
of cadmium (II) 49

Chromatography 9
thin layer 25, 32, 64

Compounds with metal-metal bond 31, 39, 49, 50, 84, 89, 161, 166

Cyclopentadienyl ligand in complexes
lanthanides 53
molybdenum 67
tungsten 74
manganese 88

197